W9-BXW-549

HOW TO BECOME A MEDICAL TRANSCRIPTIONIST

A Career for the 21st Century

HOW TO BECOME A MEDICAL TRANSCRIPTIONIST

A Career for the 21st Century

George Morton, CMT

Medical Language Development
Spring Valley, California

How to Become A Medical Transcriptionist:

A Career for the 21st Century

Copyright © 1998 by George Morton, CMT

Manufactured in the United States of America

All rights reserved. No portion of this book may be repro-
duced or transmitted in any form or by any means, electronic
or mechanical, including photocopying, recording, or by an
information storage and retrieval system, without prior
written consent of the copyright holder. Requests for permission should be made to Medical Language Development,
4122 Cortez Way, Spring Valley, California 91977.

ISBN: 0-9663470-0-5

Library of Congress Catalog Card Number: 98-96009

Published by:

Medical Language Development

4122 Cortez Way

Spring Valley, CA 91977

HARRISON COUNTY
PUBLIC LIBRARY
105 North Capitol Ave.
Corydon, IN 47112

This book is dedicated to all my students,

from whom I learn so much.

HARRISON COUNTY
PUBLIC LIBRARY
105 North Capitol Ave.
Corydon, IN 47112

*T*HANKS

*T*his book would not have been possible without the help and encouragement of so many people. First, there are those whose strength and confidence have helped me realize my own potential: my ever patient wife, Donna; Marcy Diehl of Grossmont College; and Pat Forbis of AAMT.

Deborah Ivanoff has done a beautiful job with the design and layout of this book. Chris Davis did an excellent cover design. Others who generously gave time and advice on this project were Donna Reeve-Morton, Jonathan Parker, Gloria Clanin, and Jerry Schad.

Riccy Velde and Steve Farrington were very helpful as the representatives of KNI Printers.

Thank you all.

Contents

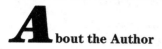

A **bout the Author**

Chapter 9

The AAMT and Professionalism

*Our network — Strength in numbers — What
the AAMT can do for you — What the AAMT can
do for our profession as a whole*

Chapter 10

Is There a Future in Medical Transcription?

*Medical transcriptionists are in demand — Will
there be too many medical transcriptionists? —
Concerns for the future — Overseas services —
Speech recognition technology — Other new
technologies*

A Few Words To You from
Successful Medical Transcriptionists

*Successful medical transcriptionists share
words of wisdom from their years of experience
— Interview with a recent medical transcription student*

ABOUT THE AUTHOR

George Morton, CMT, is a certified medical transcriptionist who has worked in the profession for 20 years. For much of
that time he operated a very successful medical transcription
service from his home, with major hospitals among his clients.

He has taught medical transcription, advanced medical
transcription, and medical terminology at Grossmont College,
El Cajon, California, since 1990.

He has introduced thousands to the profession through his
popular career-information seminars, "How To Become A
Medical Transcriptionist."

He is an active member of the American Association for
Medical Transcription and has written educational articles
for their professional journal and many other publications.
He is frequently a guest speaker at professional conferences
and symposiums.

He has represented his profession in the Healthcare
Standards Review Committee, a federal government program
to define employment skills and standards for employers and
educators.

He is owner of Medical Language Development, an education
service for professionals in healthcare, law, and insurance.

His ongoing goal throughout has been to bring to the
medical transcription profession the recognition and respect
that it deserves.

1

WHAT'S THE BIG DEAL ABOUT MEDICAL TRANSCRIPTION?

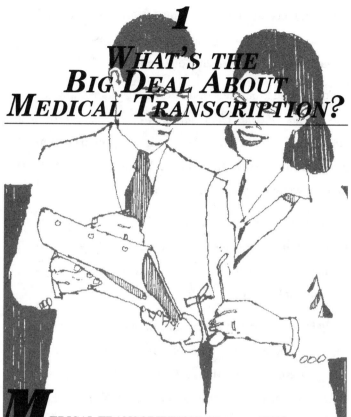

MEDICAL TRANSCRIPTION! The new HOT career!
Big demand! A great home business! Make money at home
typing for doctors! Work part-time while caring for your kids.
A job you can do on your laptop computer, sitting beside
your swimming pool!

Wow!
— ♦ —

Sounds good, doesn't it? Too good to be true? Did you
read some glossy advertising material for a medical transcription course? Saw something snazzy on the Internet? Or did
you attend a "free" seminar where they tried to sell you
hundreds or thousands of dollars' worth of classes or tapes?

Would you like some *real information* about medical transcription? From a medical transcriptionist rather than a salesperson? Yes, I thought you would.

For me and thousands of other medical transcriptionists, this is a *fascinating, challenging, stimulating, and rewarding* career. Yes, there is a demand for *good* medical transcriptionists. Yes, it can be a great home business. As for the laptop/swimming pool scenario, well....

But it takes time and hard work. Not to mention a number of other important skills not emphasized in the sales talk, such as.... Well, read this book and find out. A career like this cannot be summarized in just a few paragraphs.

My career information seminars on medical transcription have been popular for many years because the public is hungry for *facts* about this great career instead of hype and lightweight articles in "entrepreneurial" magazines. Facts from someone who's been a medical transcriptionist for 20 years. Someone who's "been there and done that." (And is still doing it.) Someone who's going to tell you what's *good and bad* about medical transcription.

This book is simply an extension of the seminar to bring this information to a wider audience.

Questions

Here are some questions I'm commonly asked:

- Is medical transcription all it's cracked up to be?

- Is it a good home business for a mother with children?

- Is there much money to be made for a good entrepreneur?

- Would it be a good part-time retirement income?

- Can I work at home but not have to run a business?

- I've worked as a nurse for many years. Will I find medical transcription easy?

- How come the ads ask only for experienced people?

- What exactly is medical transcription anyway?

- How long does it take to become a medical transcriptionist?

- Is there a future in it?

- What about speech-recognition computers?

A lot of questions. You'll find the answers in this book.

Know what you're getting into

**Take it
seriously**
_ ♦ _

This book is designed to help you make an informed decision. Are you that special kind of person who could do this work and enjoy it?

A major career decision like this should not be taken lightly.

Too many people waste a lot of time, money, and frustration in medical transcription training, only to find that the course is inadequate, or that this is simply not the right career choice for them. Please don't make these expensive mistakes.

Some of you, after reading this book, may decide that medical transcription is *not* right for you. Your small investment in this book may save you hundreds or thousands of dollars, and months or years of frustration and wasted time.

Others, after reading this book, will *know* that medical transcription is the right career choice. You'll thank me for guiding you towards a fascinating, challenging, stimulating, and rewarding profession.

Check it out.

2

WHAT IS A MEDICAL TRANSCRIPTIONIST?

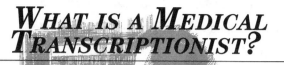

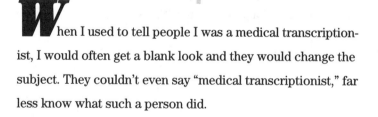

When I used to tell people I was a medical transcriptionist, I would often get a blank look and they would change the
subject. They couldn't even say "medical transcriptionist," far
less know what such a person did.

**A medical
what?**

– ♦ –

The profession is better known today, what with all the
heavy advertising of medical transcription education: "Make
easy money at home in your spare time," or words to that
effect. But the sales material gives very little idea of what
medical transcription is all about—and certainly not the
whole picture.

So, what *is* a medical transcriptionist?

Definitions

This is how the American Association for Medical Transcription defines a medical transcriptionist in its "Model Job Description":

**A medical
language
specialist**
— ♦ —

A medical language specialist who interprets and transcribes dictation by physicians and other healthcare professionals regarding patient assessment, workup, therapeutic procedures, clinical course, diagnosis, prognosis, etc. in order to document patient care and facilitate delivery of healthcare services. [Reprinted with permission. © 1990 American Association for Medical Transcription]

Does that sound a little technical? This is *my* definition:

**A patient,
intelligent
human being**
— ♦ —

A medical transcriptionist is a patient, intelligent human being who—with keen ears, quick brain, nimble fingers, and a vast knowledge of medicine, medical language, and English language—turns haphazard medical dictation into clear, legible and accurate medicolegal documents.

How Is Medical Transcription Done?

By law, every patient-doctor interaction must be documented. Not to mention that it's obviously good medical care to do so. Whether that interaction is a one-minute telephone conversation or a 16-hour heart and lung transplant, every detail must be recorded in the report. It's also medically and legally important that these reports be legible. (We all know about doctors' handwriting!) It's the job of the medical transcriptionist to turn the report into a clear and legible printed document.

Although technology has brought many changes to medical transcription, the basic process of documentation remains the same: Immediately after the patient contact, the doctor or healthcare professional picks up a telephone or microphone and dictates the medical information. It is recorded onto an audio tape or computer chip (digital recording). The medical transcriptionist plays back the recording and—via the keen ears, etc. described in my definition above—converts the spoken information into a permanent printed record—a neat and accurate typewritten report to be placed in the patient's medical chart. It may also be stored as pages of text in a "computerized patient record." (see Chapter 10)

This system of dictation and transcription is quickest and easiest for the doctor, who can then move right on to treating the next patient—leaving the paperwork/computer work to a skilled medical transcriptionist. The doctor's expensive time need not be wasted on medical documentation that can be much better and more quickly performed by a suitably trained (and less expensive) medical transcriptionist.

Accuracy

My definition of a medical transcriptionist highlights the word "accurate"—a very important word. You've read the stories about patients having the wrong leg amputated, or being given a fatal dose of medication. The documents we produce *must* be accurate. Patients' lives are at stake. Malpractice lawyers are lurking around every corner. A lot of the responsibility for accurate medical documentation rests with the medical transcriptionist—far more than we're given credit for.

The dictation is rarely 100% accurate. It's usually done in a hurry and contains both grammatical and medical mistakes. The medical transcriptionist is a physician and surgeon of language. We dissect words and phrases to understand their meaning. We understand the anatomy and physiology of the human body. We know the doctor made a mistake when she spoke about the metacarpophalangeal joint in the left foot. We know that the 300 mg (milligrams) of Synthroid the doctor dictated would cause the patient some serious medi-

Do doctors make mistakes?

− ♦ −

cal problems, and we would confirm with her that she meant to say 300 mcg (micrograms).

We understand the anatomy and physiology of the English language, so that when dictation comes to us in an unhealthy, damaged, or abused condition—full of grammatical errors and slurred words—we can repair it and make it healthy. And accurate!

Let's dissect the word "transcribe." It comes from the Latin words "across" and "write". The medical transcriptionist produces a printed document from the spoken word ("writing across" from the spoken word to the printed page).

Medicolegal Documents

My definition of a medical transcriptionist says we produce medicolegal documents. What is medicolegal? It means that as well as being a *medical* record—vital to the patient's care— it is a *legal* record. It must comply with state, federal, and even international regulations. It has to be able to stand up to court scrutiny. It may be reviewed not only by medical personnel but by lawyers, judges, insurance companies, or government officers.

Medical transcriptionists know the legal requirements for the reports they transcribe—who owns the reports, who has legal access to them, confidentiality rules, and legal guide-lines as to form and how the data should be documented.

What Medicolegal
Documents does the MT Transcribe?

As I said earlier, the report we transcribe may be a multi-page, detail-by-detail description of a 16-hour surgery. Or it may be a two-sentence notation of what was said in a follow-up telephone call with the patient. Any patient-doctor interaction must be documented.

Here are some of the reports a medical transcriptionist transcribes:

History and Physical Examination: Whenever a patient is admitted to hospital, a History and Physical Examination report (H&P) must be generated. And it needs to be on the chart right away (within an hour or two at most). Medical personnel need to know their patient, and this report contains the complete medical picture. This report may also be done on an outpatient basis when a patient is seeing a new doctor for the first time, or when a patient is undergoing an annual "checkup" or the required "physical" when applying for a new job.

Consultation: A specialist may be called in to examine a patient from a cardiovascular standpoint, or psychiatric, or urologic, or any particular medical point of view. A patient admitted to hospital for a heart attack may be diabetic, in which case the admitting physician may ask a cardiologist and an endocrinologist for a consultation. If a patient is being followed for pregnancy and is suffering from anorexia, a psychiatrist may be consulted, who will then examine the patient from that particular medical standpoint and generate a consultation report.

Discharge Summary: Whenever a patient leaves the hospital, there needs to be a discharge summary, summarizing the patient's hospital care, all the procedures carried out, all the lab test results, and with recommendations for future care.

Operative Note: Any surgical procedure, major or minor, requires an "operative report" or "procedure note." Every detail will be recorded, including the types of suture material used, the amount of blood loss, the names of each nerve and muscle encountered, and the names of the surgical instruments used. (There are many, and the medical transcriptionist is familiar with hundreds of them.)

Autopsy: Postmortem examinations are detailed and lengthy. Every part of the body is examined in detail. It's medically and legally vital to know the precise cause(s) of death, and this is the last chance to do it!

Radiology Report: Every x-ray taken has to be "read" by an M.D., usually a radiologist, with a formal report dictated and transcribed. Every technical detail needs to be discussed in this valuable diagnostic procedure. MRI and CAT scans are also reported on by the radiologist.

Pathology Report: Amputated limbs, minute skin cancers, bone marrow samples, removed appendices, biopsied tissue, etc. are sent for formal examination by an M.D. pathologist, who generates a detailed report.

Other: Workers Compensation reports, Social Security evaluations, medical correspondence to lawyers or insurance companies, social service evaluations, psychological testing reports, chart notes, progress notes, and emergency room notes are some of the other documents a medical transcriptionist will transcribe.

Although chart notes, progress notes, and ER notes are still sometimes handwritten, the days of handwritten medical reports are coming to an end. The information is too valuable to be illegible. Lives depend on it. Lawyers and insurance companies are insisting on typed reports, as are the medical personnel who have to read them!

A Medical Transcriptionist is Not a Typist

Don't ever call a medical transcriptionist a typist.

Creative keyboard artists
— ♦ —

There are many skilled professionals who use keyboards in their work — court reporters, authors, computer programmers, concert pianists. They are paid for the skill and experience that go behind each keystroke. Likewise the medical transcriptionist. This is not copy typing. There's complex intellectual work going on here.

If our job were simply typing, then, at a modest speed of 70 wpm, we would produce 3000+ full lines of text per eight-hour shift (allowing for the usual breaks). As it is, most transcriptionists would be happy to produce 1500 lines on a good day. Which suggests that there is a lot more to our work than just typing!

Even slow typists—competent in all the other medical transcription skills—can be high producers. I am a good example of that. The fastest typing speed test I ever passed was 65 wpm, and that was a struggle. Yet, my quantity of production, wherever I've worked, has always been above the office average. Because I'm hot stuff at all the other components of medical transcription (excuse my modesty). And the *quality* of my work is something of which I've always been proud.

So What Goes on Between the Keystrokes?

The medical transcriptionist is performing a complex mental process that involves listening, thinking, translating, and interpreting, using an immense data base of medical knowledge and English language skill—a process, by the way, that cannot be replicated by any computer (see Speech Recognition Technology, Chapter 10).

Brain power
– ♦ –

The following examples demonstrate this well:

1.   These three phrases sound identical to each other. A "typist," untrained in medical transcription, might hear

and type any one of the following. They sound the same in rapid dictation:

"...and effusion at the L5S1 inner space."

"...and diffusion at the L5S1 interspace."

"...and a fusion at the L5-S1 interspace."

The medical transcriptionist knows—from her knowledge of medicine—that only the third of these is correct.

2. A typist untrained in medical transcription hears: "Prednisone was reduced 2.5 mg." The medical transcriptionist hears the same thing and thinks, "This could be 'reduced 2.5 mg' or 'reduced to 0.5 mg.'" Either could be correct. The medical transcriptionist checks the chart or confirms it with the doctor. Prednisone dosages are a serious matter and not to be guessed.

3. A typist, transcribing verbatim, might type: "Mr. Smith had a cabbage in 1993." The medical transcriptionist, however, would transcribe: "Mr. Smith had a coronary artery bypass graft in 1993." Doctors have an annoying habit of abbreviating everything, and CABG (they pronounce it "cabbage"), for coronary artery bypass graft, is one of those abbreviations. For obvious legal reasons, abbreviations are generally not acceptable in medical reports, except for a few that are widely used and understood. After all, an abbreviation can have any number of interpretations. Who knows which one the doctor meant?

HARRISON COUNTY
PUBLIC LIBRARY
105 North Capitol Ave.
Corydon, IN 47112

4.   The doctor dictates: "The patient is to take 25 mg of digoxin each morning." The medical transcriptionist recognizes that the doctor made an error in dictation, and changes it to "0.25 mg of digoxin," *with a note to the doctor* to confirm any change or correction.

These are just a few obvious examples showing the knowledge and judgment constantly used by the medical transcriptionist. There are thousands more, sometimes just little words or inflexions of sound that can make a big difference to these medicolegal documents.

The Medical Language Specialist

The medical transcriptionist is knowledgeable in the vast, complex, and ever-changing field of medicine. The medical transcriptionist is familiar with what goes on in an inguinal hernia repair, an arthroscopy, a cesarean section, a retinal detachment repair, and hundreds of other medical procedures. The medical transcriptionist is familiar with the slang terms used, knows what most of the abbreviations stand for, knows the brand names of the surgical instruments, knows how to spell long drug names, and knows how to research new and unfamiliar material. The medical transcriptionist does not balk at hearing a mumble that sounds like "the shelving edge of Poupart's ligament," or "bleeders were coagulated with the Bovie," or "the Minnesota Multiphasic Personality Inventory."

Medical
knowledge
— ◆ —

HARRISON COUNTY
PUBLIC LIBRARY

Continuing Education

Medicine is growing by leaps and bounds. The medical transcriptionist must keep up with all the latest medical developments, or pretty soon her skills are obsolete. We attend medical lectures and read medical journals. How can we ensure an accurate report if we don't know what the doctor is talking about?

Continuing education is part of the job for a medical transcriptionist.

Our Skills are Respected

The doctor knows that the medical transcriptionist will surgically repair poor grammar and sloppy sentences and produce a report that is accurate and professional. The doctor will usually sign the report without even reading it — such is the degree of trust and responsibility accorded the medical transcriptionist.

Every medical transcriptionist will tell you that when a doctor is kind enough to spell a "difficult" word for us in the dictation, that spelling will be wrong more than 50% of the time! (That's not an exaggeration.) Just leave it up to us, doctor, thank you very much.

We're important!
− ♦ −

Can you see why medical transcriptionists take pride in their skills and call themselves *professionals* and *medical language specialists*?

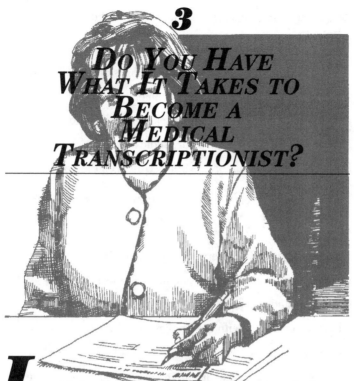

3

DO YOU HAVE WHAT IT TAKES TO BECOME A MEDICAL TRANSCRIPTIONIST?

I've said already that not just anyone can do medical transcription. Here are eleven skills and character attributes you will need if you wish to succeed as a medical transcriptionist. You should consider them carefully before you invest a lot of time, money, and energy in pursuing this career. Good medical transcriptionists are in demand because this is such a rare combination of skills.

Skill #1: A Love of Language

Are you a "word nerd?" Do you like to read? Do you enjoy crossword puzzles? Enjoy spelling bees? Are you always looking up words to learn their meanings and derivations? Do you enjoy good literature?

Did you take and enjoy foreign languages at school? Were you good at English? (Not just capable, but *good*.) Can you punctuate and repair ungrammatical sentences and poorly spoken English? Try "Test Your Medical Transcription Potential " at the back of this book. How well did you do?

Fact: A high level of English language competency is the medical transcriptionist's most important skill.

You thought medical terminology and typing speed were the most important skills? While not unimportant, these skills can be learned by most people with a little time and persistence. Competency with the English language, however, is something more special. It is acquired gradually over many years. A lot of otherwise bright and successful people never seem to be able to master it.

The medical transcription student should start out with at least some English language proficiency—and certainly a love of language. A good medical transcription course will include further study in this area, perhaps a class called Business English or English Fundamentals, where grammar, punctuation, and sentence structure are emphasized. A student who needs to develop these skills should do a lot more reading (good literature and medical journals, not the National Enquirer).

Warning: Students without good language skills have a hard time in medical transcription classes.

Not only are we medical language specialists. I prefer an even broader term: "language specialists."

Why is this so important? Remember, these are *medicolegal* documents. Careless punctuation and misused words can make a serious difference to the meaning of a sentence, resulting in possible medical problems for the patient and/or legal problems for the doctor. Even if the consequences are not so dire, there remains a need for accuracy and quality in transcription to maintain the healthcare provider's professional status.

The dictating doctors will seldom provide correct punctuation and grammar for you. This is *your* skill, what *you* have been trained in. They trust *you* to take care of it for them. Doctors can make the blind see, the lame walk, and restore a dying heart. But punctuation and good English? Well...

Some doctors, particularly those with English as a second language, will specifically request that you improve their dictation to make them look and sound professional. What a responsibility! Not only does this require considerable skill with language, but you need a good knowledge of medicine to ensure that the medical meaning remains intact and accurate.

**Help
doctors
look
professional**
– ♦ –

How they teach punctuation at medical school

Period   = the monthly menstrual cycle

Comma   = a state of unconsciousness

Colon   = part of the digestive tract

Skill #2: A Genuine Interest In Medicine

Do you really enjoy this stuff? Are you absolutely fascinated by medical science? For some people, gallbladders and hernias and runny noses can get pretty boring unless you have a genuine interest in medicine. Keeping up with all the latest developments and procedures is fascinating for me, as well as a challenge that I enjoy. It should be the same for you. You're going to learn a lot about medicine as a medical transcriptionist.

Skill #3: Comfort with Medical Terminology

Believe it or not, after just one semester of medical terminology, you'll have a medical vocabulary of thousands of the most widely used medical terms. Here are some common medical words. Do they frighten you? They're long and ugly, but relatively easy to figure out, once you know how. Let's get our scalpels and dissect them:

Hystero/salpingo/-oophor/ectomy

You may recognize the last part of this word: "-ectomy." Know any other words with this ending? Tonsillectomy?

Adenoidectomy? Appendectomy? Yes, "-ectomy" means surgical removal.

The word parts "hystero," "salpingo," and "oophoro" mean uterus, (Fallopian) tubes, and ovaries respectively. So figure out what hysterosalpingo-oophorectomy means.

Uvulo/palato/pharyngo/plasty

Another common medical suffix is "-plasty." It means surgical repair. As in plastic surgery. In this case we have a repair of the uvula, which is that little flap of tissue hanging down at the back of your throat (uvula is the Latin word for a bunch of grapes, which the tissue resembles); the palate, which is the roof of your mouth; and the pharynx, which is the upper area of your throat. A uvulopalatopharyngoplasty is a surgical repair procedure that may be done to remove excess tissue that forms in this area. The excess tissue can interfere with breathing when you sleep, causing sleep apnea (a/pnea = "without breathing").

What would hysteroplasty mean?

Chole/docho/jejun/ostomy

The suffix "-ostomy" means "a new opening." (A col/ostomy is a new opening surgically created in the colon.) "Chole-" means bile or gall (a digestive substance stored in the gall-bladder). "Docho-" means a duct or channel. "Jejuno-" pertains to a part of the small intestine called the jejunum. A choledochojejunostomy, therefore, is the surgical creation of a new opening between the bile duct and the small intestine.

There are tens of thousands of medical words, and new ones being coined every day. No one can possibly know them all. Even the most experienced medical transcriptionist is constantly looking up words — confirming a spelling or a meaning. Knowing where to look, and how to use the reference books, is an important part of the job. It's a skill you begin to develop in class and continue to develop for the rest of your career. You become a Sherlock Holmes, trying to interpret an unusual dictated sound into a correctly spelled word that makes sense in the context. The vast and complex structure of your knowledge of medical terminology, anatomy, and physiology is like Gaudi's cathedral in Barcelona. It's always being added to, and never complete.

A word detective
– ♦ –

Skill #4: Listening Skills

Do you need to have good hearing to be a medical transcriptionist? My hearing has always been borderline. But this has never held me back in medical transcription. It may actually have helped, because it's made my listening skills more acute. I've learned to interpret incomplete or unclear sounds to make sense of them. I've learned the art of "auditory processing." (That's neuropsychology jargon.)

This auditory processing is very much a skill of the medical transcriptionist. A skill that develops gradually as you train. It's interesting to see some students doing so well in every other aspect of their medical transcription education, yet having a great deal of difficulty interpreting the sounds they hear—medical words or otherwise.

The small words are the tricky ones. Words like "and," "an," "in," , and the prefix "un-" are easily confused because they are often mumbled or not said at all; a wrong interpretation can result in major differences to the meaning of a sentence. "If" and "of" often sound the same. "15" and "50" sound the same. "Tearful" and "cheerful" sound the same. Believe it or not, the words "two" and "three" often sound very similar in dictation. The consonants "b" and "v" usually sound identical, as do the consonants "s" and "f." The prefixes "hyper-" and "hypo-" are often indistinguishable, yet they have opposite meanings. No guessing please—someone's life may be at stake. Get to work, Sherlock.

The long medical words are actually easier to understand than the little English words. They have more "hooks" for your brain to catch onto, more auditory clues.

Listening skills don't develop overnight. They're one of the main reasons why you can't become a medical transcriptionist in four months or eight months. The vast terminology of medicine may be dictated in an infinite number of permutations, with varying pronunciation, carelessly, ungrammatically, with slang, jargon, abbreviations, regional and foreign accents, poorly recorded, etc., etc. That's why you'll need to spend 12 to 18 months on your education before you're ready for that entry-level position in medical transcription.

Skill #5 A Professional Attitude

The medical transcriptionist plays a vital role in healthcare. With a broad knowledge of medical terminology, medical procedures, anatomy, physiology, pharmacology, medical records regulations, pathophysiology, computer skills, auditory skills, English language, grammar, and punctuation, the medical transcriptionist deserves *respect* (and a much higher salary!) for this unique combination of skills. The doctors couldn't do it. The nurses couldn't do it. Medical records department managers couldn't do it. Someone with Ph.D.'s in English, Anatomy, and Physiology couldn't do it. Speech recognition computers couldn't do it. Only the medical transcriptionist can do this work.

As a competent, skilled medical transcriptionist, you have a lot to be proud of. We are *professionals* and nothing less. This professionalism is reflected in the work of a good medical transcriptionist. (See Chapter 9)

Skill #6 The Ability To Work Under Pressure

Being vital to good patient care, the reports we generate are needed promptly by our fellow healthcare professionals. STAT (immediately) is a word you're going to hear a lot as a medical transcriptionist.

For example, when a patient is admitted to hospital, there must be an admission History and Physical Examination report on the chart almost immediately. A surgeon cannot operate without that report.

In my earlier days as a medical transcriptionist, I sometimes worked alone on the late evening shift at a particular hospital. If a patient was admitted for emergency surgery, perhaps the victim of an automobile accident or a stabbing, a very quick process would ensue: The doctor, having just examined the patient in the emergency room, would dictate the History and Physical Examination report. I would transcribe the report the instant it had been recorded. I would print it out (praying that the printer was working tonight), then literally run down to the surgery suite to deliver it by hand to the waiting surgeon, who was gloved and masked and anxious to read this important information on the person about to be operated on.

True story
– ♦ –

The need for such quick turnaround on reports is not always quite so acute, but there is definitely *time pressure* involved in our work.

There's another reason for medical reports to be produced promptly: The doctor or hospital won't get reimbursed by the insurance companies without them!

Some doctors are notorious for procrastinating with their dictation. Which puts even more time pressure on the transcriptionist! If you plan to become self-employed in this field, be prepared for Dr. Procrastinator to call at 8:00 p.m. on

Dr. Procrastinator
– ♦ –

Sunday night with a stack of dictation that's needed for tomorrow morning!

Time pressure is also an element in medical transcription inasmuch as many of us are paid according to *how much* we produce in a given time period (piecework). We (or our employers) may put pressure on ourselves to produce more in those situations, often at the expense of quality and accuracy and our own health. (see Chapter 5)

Skill #7: Perfectionism

If you haven't realized it by now, the medical transcriptionist needs to be a perfectionist. I've already stressed the importance of accuracy in our work, and the reasons for it. It's not enough to guess at words, or to transcribe what you *think* you heard. Someone's life may depend on it. If you were a hospital patient, would you like *your* medical reports to be full of guesses and inaccuracies?

If a word or phrase is not clear, is ambiguous, or is something that may have been dictated in error, the transcriptionist will leave a blank space and attach a note for the doctor to provide the correct word(s). A report with such blank spaces is still a legal document. Whereas a report with guesses and text that makes no sense belongs in the trash. It probably would be thrown out of court in any legal situation.

A good medical transcriptionist is a perfectionist.

Skill #8: Patience

You'll need patience from the outset. You can only learn by practice, practice, practice—listening to hours and hours of dictation. You can be job-ready in a year or less if you have the luxury of many free hours a day to practice, some good material to practice with, a good instructor, and a lot of patience. Most of us need a little longer.

You'll need patience on the job. Doctors aren't the easiest people to work with. They're always in a hurry, and the milliseconds they save by not punching in the correct dictation codes or patient numbers, or by dictating at a thoughtlessly fast speed, or abbreviating every second phrase, can cause many minutes of wasted time for the transcriptionist.

The doctor has the patients. The medical transcriptionist has the patience.

Skill #9: Integrity

Sssshhh..... Medical reports can be full of juicy gossip. DON'T BLAB! It's quite likely you will come across a report on someone you know personally or someone well known in the community. Or a patient with an embarrassing or "funny" problem. It should not need to be emphasized that the information you are dealing with is *private and confidential.* Your employer may have you sign a contract to ensure that you understand this; but whether or not you sign such a

Confidentiality
— ◆ —

document, a breach of confidentiality may mean the end of your career in the medical field.

Integrity also ties in with the perfectionism we looked at earlier. We want our work to be perfect not only for our own pride, but also for the fact that our patients deserve the best possible medical care, which will be served by conscientious medical transcription.

Skill #10: A Love of Learning

As a medical transcriptionist, your education doesn't finish when you leave school. It's only just begun! Every report transcribed is an education for the medical transcriptionist, another brick in the mighty cathedral of knowledge.

We're always learning
– ◆ –

A successful medical transcriptionist enjoys the continuing education that is an integral part of the job. We learn by attending medical lectures and presentations. We learn by reading articles in the newspapers and professional journals. Our local cable TV company may have a medical channel. A well-educated and informed medical transcriptionist has a competitive edge in the workplace. And one who does *not* keep up will soon be obsolete.

If you think learning is a chore, then medical transcription may not be for you. Because it's part of the job.

Skill #11: Independence

Do you need a lot of social interaction in your working day? If so, medical transcription may not be your cup of tea.

But if you can sit and work independently at your computer for eight hours a day, giving each report your best attention and concentration, and giving each patient your conscientious best effort, then you have one of the skills of a successful medical transcriptionist.

Not that you're tied to your work station. You'll be "huddling" with your fellow transcriptionists on a difficult piece of dictation. You'll be getting up and stretching and taking those very necessary ergonomic breaks (see Chapter 5).

Certainly, there are gregarious medical transcriptionists. And you should hear the noise at our meetings and conventions! But these people know when to switch it on and switch it off.

You need to be the independent type, the kind of person who says, "I've got a very important job of work to do. It requires a lot of concentration and I don't want any interruptions."

4

SOME GOOD THINGS ABOUT MEDICAL TRANSCRIPTION

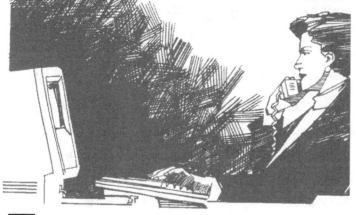

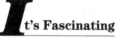t's Fascinating

The vast and wonderful world of medicine is a *fascinating* subject. Learn about the amazing human body and all the latest developments in medical science. Learn in school. Learn on the job. Even after 20 years, you'll still be learning from every report that you transcribe, and from the medical lectures you attend, and the medical articles you read. There's always something new to learn. It's great to do work that's intellectually stimulating.

> ***Warning:*** Hypochondriacs may have a difficult time in medical transcription. Think of all the things that could be wrong with you!

It's Challenging

The dictation may be full of complex terminology, jargon, abbreviations, and mistakes spoken at 100 miles per hour in a foreign accent. Yet it's taken for granted that a clear and accurate medical document will appear on the chart in record time! Some of us enjoy that challenge. We thrive on it!

It's Rewarding

**The MT
is a VIP**

– ♦ –

It's professionally rewarding to know that, as a medical transcriptionist, you play a vital role in the nation's health care. As I said in the previous chapter, we are given a lot of trust and responsibility for the quality and accuracy of our work. Most doctors are very aware of this, even if they sometimes forget to show their gratitude. As a medical transcriptionist, you have a skill that very few are capable of. You are a professional and have professional satisfaction in your work. The people of this country couldn't live (literally) without prompt, skilled, and accurate medical documentation.

What about financial rewards? A good, experienced medical transcriptionist can make a decent living in this business. (See Chapter 6 for rates of pay). If you're a good business person on top of that, you can do very well financially. Here's how, in a nutshell:

Train hard. Get lots of work experience. Start a business. Do a great job. Gain a good reputation. Get flooded with work. Hire more and more subcontractors or employees. Be a good manager and good business person, as well as a good medical transcriptionist. And get rich!

Easier said than done; but a few smart medical transcriptionists have succeeded in this way.

It Can be Quite Entertaining!

Of course, *you* won't be the new transcriptionist who transcribes, "The patient had a baloney amputation." But some have made this lovely goof, which actually should be transcribed as, "The patient had a below-knee amputation."

And if you're starting in the pathology lab, you will know that the specimen sent for the pathologist's examination is not "skinny lips" but "skin ellipse."

Our professional journals and newsletters constantly feature the latest "bloopers." Needless to say, nine times out of ten, they originate with the doctor rather than the transcriptionist. Here are just a few examples that I've encountered:

Bloopers
– ♦ –

"The patient has a hearing aid in his right eye."

"The patient's grandmother has a history of neurological disorder, but she is currently dead."

"The patient has been depressed ever since she began seeing me in 1991." (Dictated by a particularly morose-sounding doctor.)

"She has a high IQ and is a member of Mensis."

"The patient has no current fever, although his wife said he was very hot in bed last night."

"Her memory was intact to recent and remote events. She was oriented to person, place, and time. Her memory was intact to recent and remote events."

"The patient had a hearing test last month but has not heard the results."

"The patient is a right-handed, blond-eyed, blue-haired Caucasian male."

A spellchecker I used a few years back, when they were less efficient than they are now, did not recognize the drug Micronase that had been prescribed for a diabetic patient. The spellchecker instead came up with the helpful suggestion of "macaroons."

It's Mobile

Where would you like to retire?

— ♦ —

What a mobile profession! Wherever there are patients and doctors, there are medical transcriptionists. We're in demand wherever we go. Demand seems to be fairly level around the country. So if your spouse is transferred, or you'd like to move to a different part of the country, you can very easily take your portable medical transcription skill with you and be in equal demand in your new location.

In this new age of telecommunication, you can even retire to your little mountain cabin in Vermont or your beach house in Hawaii and be a part-time medical transcriptionist. Information, including the recorded human voice and word processing text, can now be transferred freely and quickly around the world from computer to computer via telephone line. You can have digitally recorded dictation "zapped" to your cabin or beach house via modem. You can then digitally "zap" the completed transcript via modem back to the originator. Not a cassette tape or a piece of paper in sight at your end of the operation.

Telecommunication is the trend in this industry. More and more home-based transcriptionists, whether employed or self-employed, are receiving and transmitting their work from home. (See Chapter 6 for more information about the transcription workplace.)

It's Flexible

Work at home. Start your own business. Work at a big hospital. Work for a transcription service. Work at your family doctor's office. There are quite a number of work settings available for the medical transcriptionist. (See

What hours would you like?
— ♦ —

Chapter 6). In most of these settings, you can work full-time, part-time, overtime, per diem, on call, graveyard shift, morning shift, evening shift, Saturdays through Wednesdays, weekends only, or any combination thereof. It's usually possible to work out a work schedule to fit your lifestyle. Hospital transcription departments usually work around the clock, seven days a week. As do some large transcription services. And a home-based transcriptionist can fit a work schedule around his/her daily routine.

There's No Age Limit

As we reach our more "mature" years, we tend to worry about our employability. We know we are healthy and employable at 45, 55, or 65, but how do we convince employers?

Medical transcription is well suited to mature people. And by mature, I don't necessarily mean "old." I mean someone who has some life experience.

Although we have some "wiz kids" in our classes in their late teens and early 20s, they tend to be the exception. For whatever reason, people seem to do better in this profession a little later in life when they want to change career, or after they've raised a family and want to get back into the work force.

Most employers seem to recognize this and realize that medical transcriptionists in their later years can be valuable employees. I used to work with a medical transcriptionist who worked well into her 80s. And she was sharp. This work must be good for the brain!

I've never heard of any age, sex, or race discrimination in this profession. I won't say it's not there, but if it exists, it's very rare.

It's Secure

There seems to be a lot of "job insecurity" these days. The world, its industry and technology are changing fast. We have to keep up with these changes and be ready to adapt. We don't have the same job security our parents took for granted.

When I give career-information seminars about medical transcription, I meet many bright and intelligent adults who have recently lost their jobs and feel very insecure. They have families to take care of, and their later years to plan for. Maybe the bank just kicked them out after 20 years of service, with one week's notice. No "golden handshake." No pension. Nothing. Defense and real estate are two other industries "downsizing" and supplying my seminars with people looking for a new start.

Is there more security in health care than in other careers? Certainly health care is more recession-proof. There will always be health care. There will always be a need for doctors and nurses and all the necessary support staff. But this industry is changing fast too, and there are many skills in health care that will be obsolete in a few years.

Will medical transcription become obsolete?

There will *always* be a need for documentation of medical information, whether it's stored on computer disk or paper. The medical transcriptionist is the one person with the medical knowledge and the language skills to be able to safely perform this documentation, whatever the technology. The doctor seldom has the time (at $150+ an hour!) or the language skills or the patience to accurately enter this data in whatever format is required. As we saw in Chapter 2, it's easiest, the most economical, and the least time-consuming, for the doctor to simply recite the medical information fresh from memory, knowing that the information will then be processed into an acceptable medicolegal document. The medical transcriptionist/medical language specialist will take care of it. So: job security for medical transcriptionists!

How else could it be done?

– ♦ –

Some people think speech recognition technology will take over our work. Computers can now respond to the human voice, as well as to mouse and keyboard. Please see my discussion of this in Chapter 10. It's not something we transcriptionists are worried about.

Growing population = more patients = more doctors = more medical reports = more medical transcriptionists.

Universal health care (if it ever happens) = more patients, etc.

Although I have concerns (Chapter 10) about a bigger labor pool of medical transcriptionists, the ever-growing demand should be able to absorb the extra supply. There's an old and wise saying, "There's always room at the top." Enough doctors care about quality that good medical transcriptionists will become even more sought after, especially as the skills and knowledge required become even more complex. There continue to be ads for good, experienced medical transcriptionists, with the occasional employer even offering a sign-on bonus! Yes, get $1,000 just for taking the job! I once saw a $3,000 bonus offered. It's a positive sign for the future.

Room at the top
– ♦ –

So train hard, get your experience, be better than the rest, get your CMT certification (see Chapter 7), and you'll have a secure future in medical transcription.

5
WHAT ARE THE CHALLENGES OF MEDICAL TRANSCRIPTION?

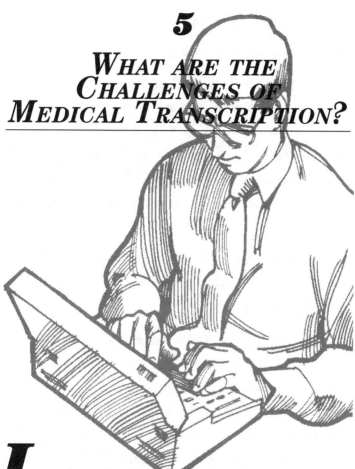

I warned you that this would not be a glossy sales pitch for medical transcription. This work has its challenges, and I want you to be well aware of them before you spend time and money on training for a career that might not suit you. What some people see as positively stimulating challenges, others may see as headaches, problems, or difficulties.

Let's look at what these challenges (or problems?) might be.

It's Physically Demanding

What? A sedentary job physically demanding? Am I joking?

A survey of medical transcriptionists will find a surprising number of physical ailments related to their work. Number one is carpal tunnel syndrome, the bane of our profession. A lot of us have it to varying degrees. Surgery does not have a high success rate with this condition. However, we're beginning to win this battle with prevention and good ergonomics (see below).

Carpal tunnel syndrome
– ◆ –

Other common physical conditions in this line of work are lower and upper back problems, neck, shoulder, and arm problems, migraines, and eye problems.

Ergonomics is the science of adapting the work environment for optimum employee health. A lot of information is now available on ergonomics, and this has become a big industry. Employers are aware that an ergonomically correct working environment is economically correct. Workers' Compensation and sick leave costs remind them of this. In the medical transcription workplace nowadays you're almost certain to find good-posture seating, good lighting, wrist rests, ergonomic keyboards, and readily available literature on ergonomics. If any of these are not provided, you will be well within your rights to insist that they are. You will be recommended, if not required, to take a five-minute break every hour, as well as the usual coffee and lunch breaks. You will actually be *more* productive by taking these breaks.

A healthy work environment
– ◆ –

It's up to you to be responsible for maintenance of your most important working tool—your body. It's easy to forget this because we really concentrate on our work and get tensed up without realizing it. Or we might be overstressing our bodies striving to reach a productivity quota. Develop your good ergonomic habits early, and this irreplaceable tool—your body—will be productive for a long time. Because when physical problems occur, they're awfully hard, or impossible, to fix.

Your most
important
tool
– ◆ –

If you have wrist, back, or eye problems even before you enter medical transcription training, get some practical advice from your physician or chiropractor.

Mental Stamina

The mental stamina required to do this work has always been the hardest part of the job for me. Eight hours (or more) per day at a computer is mentally taxing. This is high-level brain work! Each report needs your full attention and concentration. The last report of the day requires the same degree of mental effort as the first. Each patient deserves your best.

We mentioned the ergonomic need to take a five-minute break every hour. Your mental ergonomics require this break also. Tea and walking have always been my "refreshers." Even a five-minute walk every hour will keep fresh, oxygen-

Mental
ergonomics
– ◆ –

ated blood circulating around your brain cells. Many transcriptionists go for a run or a brisk walk during their lunch hour and return refreshed.

Medical transcription professionals need to be "alert and oriented" (a term the doctors like to use).

Isolation vs. Independence

What some of us would call isolation (*negative*), others would call independence (*positive*). If you're the gregarious, people-oriented sort, medical transcription might be a lonely profession. We're expected to spend the best part of eight hours daily interacting with a computer. And we really have to shut out the rest of the world while we're doing this, whether working at an office or at home.

Prison?

– ♦ –

If this sounds like self-imposed imprisonment, then you may not like the "isolation" of medical transcription.

Or freedom?

– ♦ –

If it sounds like freedom from mindless chatter and office politics, then you'll appreciate the "independence" of medical transcription.

Most Dictation Is Not Good Dictation.

Paperwork and dictation are usually *the last thing* a doctor wants to do. They're put off until the last minute, and then done rather hastily.

Great dictators I have known

Maybe about 20% of the doctors dictate clearly and conscientiously. About 70% will give you some pretty mediocre dictation, a mistake here and there, but nothing we can't handle without a good education and a little patience. The remaining 10% are just plain awful. They will dictate at record-breaking speed because they've dictated this routine report a thousand times before. The words will be slurred and indistinct. They will dictate while eating. (They don't realize that our ears are as close to that intimate chomping sound as the microphone is to their mouths. Sometimes we have to pick food crumbs out of our ears.)

A doctor may dictate while driving. All sorts of special-effects sounds there. A doctor may dictate in the emergency room—a noisy, bustling place—with the screams of a woman in labor very prominent. A doctor may dictate in the newborn nursery. WAAAHH x 25! A microphone or telephone mouthpiece may drift slowly away from the dictating mouth while a chart is being flipped through; we hear loud rustling paper and a faint voice in the background. There may be static on the telephone line—which may not sound loud to the dictator, but it amplifies awfully on the recording. Sometimes the recording equipment is faulty, causing extraneous noise or dropped words. There are many foreign doctors in this country. Some have a hard time with the English language. And there are American doctors who have a hard time with the English language.

Special effects

– ♦ –

It's all in a day's work for the medical transcriptionist—
who gets great satisfaction in deciphering a tricky word or
phrase. And if we can't decipher it, a "huddle" of us surely
will. Would this be a stimulating challenge for you, or a
problem?

The Longest Sentence I Ever Served

Dr. X. is famous for serving us with long sentences. I think
this one qualifies for the Guinness Book of Records:

> *"This is the first psychiatrist medication evalu-*
> *ation for a 57-year-old State Disability-disabled*
> *computer analyst, who has 30 years' service*
> *with a company contracting with the City of*
> *San Diego, because of amyloid angiopathy, in*
> *which he presented in December 1993 with a*
> *left temporal stroke with a major deficit, in that*
> *he couldn't figure out how to sign on to his*
> *computer terminal, and then somewhat recov-*
> *ered from this and was able to return to work*
> *until it recurred in June 1995, at which time he*
> *underwent neurosurgical exploration of his left*
> *temporal lobe and had evacuation of a clot by*
> *Dr. M., together with biopsy of the wall of his*
> *temporal lobe at the site of bleeding, and this*
> *came back as showing amyloid angiopathy."*

What did I do with this gem of dictation? After all, the medical transcriptionist is trained to change nothing in the dictation unless it is grammatically or medically wrong. And we must confirm the change with the dictating doctor unless we're 110% sure of our correction. Even if the dictation sounds awkward, or is something less than a literary work of art, we should leave it alone if it's grammatically and medically correct. We are trained to limit our editing because there's a risk that we might unknowingly change the *meaning* of the dictation.

Careful editing

– ♦ –

Dr. X's sentence isn't exactly wrong. I think the punctuation I've given it here is grammatically correct. But to save the reader of the report from a big headache, I transcribed it in three sentences instead of one, with no change to the meaning. I put a period after the first "angiopathy." I then omitted the words "in which" and began a new sentence at "He presented..." I put a period after "1995" and began a new sentence, "At *that* time he underwent..."

Having worked for Dr. X. for many years now, he's given me license to make him sound a little more professional. Many doctors (especially the foreign ones), once they get to know you and respect your skills, will ask you to make them "look good" on paper.

The medical transcriptionist edits only with caution and experience.

It Can Be Stressful

We read in Chapter 2 about time pressure in our work—knowing how important it is that reports get on the charts promptly, and how every minute counts. Some people thrive (*positive*) on this kind of pressure. For others, it's just plain stressful (*negative*).

Burnout
– ♦ –

We mentioned the stress of a production-oriented work environment (more pay for more lines of text transcribed). It's important that the medical transcriptionist not burn herself out in this kind of environment by trying to make a few extra dollars. Otherwise those few extra dollars may have to pay for her carpal tunnel surgery. Or her psychiatrist bills. Some employers have found that "incentive pay" actually decreases production. It certainly lowers the quality of the work. A burned-out medical transcriptionist doesn't make much money—for herself or for her employer.

I've heard of production-oriented workplaces where the transcriptionists work through their coffee and lunch breaks (by their own choice) and don't give themselves time to "huddle" with co-workers on a difficult word, or even have time to say "hello" to each other.

Healthcare by piecework?
– ♦ –

I hope medicine as a whole doesn't take this direction toward piecework. Imagine the following situations in a hospital: Can we perform one more C-section before 12 o'clock? Pay nurses bonuses for every extra patient they "care" for? The MRI lab operating like 50-Minute Foto? File clerks in Medical Records being paid according to how many charts they file? (Know the trouble a misfiled chart causes?)

There's another kind of stress that medical transcriptionists face: The information in the reports we transcribe can be distressing. There are some very sad physical and social problems described, sometimes in children. Patients die. It's hard not to become emotionally involved. Even though we don't interact with the patients directly, medical transcriptionists get to know them very intimately.

Getting Your First Job

Graduates may spend a month or two getting their first job. It may be because they don't pursue every opportunity, or because they have particular requirements. On the other hand, many students get jobs *before* they graduate. If you pursue every opportunity, you won't be long without work.

Still, where other professions welcome interns and apprentices, medical transcription employers are often too hesitant to open their arms to even the best graduate students. It's frustrating, and just plain unfair.

Students sometimes become discouraged when they read newspaper want ads that say "experience only." The students say, "You can't get a job without experience. And you can't get experience without a job."

Just remember this: If new graduates were never hired, then our profession would gradually fade and become obsolete with the death of the last "experienced" transcriptionist. It's only logical—as with any other profession—that there's an attrition rate that new transcriptionists have to fill.

Do the ads mean what they say? Many of my students have proven them wrong. They've applied anyway and shown the skills, intelligence, and enthusiasm that more "experienced" applicants did not show. So they got the job.

When the newspaper ads ask for experience, that's what they would *prefer*. Slightly less training time involved for the employer. But many employers will most certainly consider a good graduate, particularly one who's been through a good, well-reputed, comprehensive training course. Having worked with hundreds of medical transcriptionists over many years, I can safely say that some of my "inexperienced" graduates do better work than many "experienced" MTs—who may be burned out, or sloppy in their work. And savvy employers know this. Their extra time invested in grooming the graduate to a productive level is quickly rewarded with a conscientious, quality-oriented, hard worker. Even the experienced MT has a learning curve in each new work setting—getting used to new equipment, new doctors' voices, new terminology, etc.

I wish more want ads asked for *quality* rather than years of experience and high typing speeds. The latter are *not* the most important skills.

"Experience" does not mean "quality"

— ♦ —

Summary

So there you have some of the *challenges* of medical transcription. It is a challenging profession. That's why good, experienced medical transcriptionists are in demand. Medical transcriptionists—like all successful professionals—*thrive* on challenge.

6

THE MEDICAL TRANSCRIPTION WORKPLACE AND RATES OF PAY

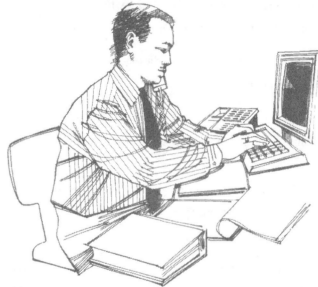

T*here are a number of work settings for the medical transcriptionist. Let's take a look at them.*

The Hospital

"Downsizing." "Outsourcing." Two words that are all too common in hospitals today. Many hospitals are reducing costs (or think they are) by having their transcription done by outside services rather than by an "in-house" transcription department. Medical transcription opportunities in hospitals are far fewer than they were just a few years ago. A pity,

In the heart of the action – ◆ –

because I always found this to be the most interesting and varied kind of work. You're right there in the heart of the action. You hear the "Code Blue" (emergency) calls over the hospital intercom. You see the doctors who dictate the reports, and might even get to know some of them.

Hospital payscales and benefits are good too—especially medical benefits!

Some hospitals—and the doctors who work in them—see value in retaining their own on-site transcription departments. Access, accountability, and quality control may be the deciding factors. Transcription employment opportunities do still exist in hospitals, but there's probably a greater demand for the fewer positions available.

A larger hospital may have separate transcription departments for general transcription, radiology transcription, pathology transcription, and emergency room transcription. Take your pick. They'll be paid the same, because you need the same all-round medical knowledge for each.

The Medical Clinic or Doctor's Office

The same "outsourcing" trend exists here, although many clinics and offices too continue to prefer on-site transcription.

Many transcriptionists enjoy this setting—working for just one doctor or a particular group of doctors—and may establish long and mutually beneficial working relationships. You may have other skills to offer this employer (medical office management, insurance billing, coding, reception, or medical assisting) and would transcribe just part of the time.

A Transcription Service

Transcription services vary in size from large national corporations employing hundreds, to small, one-person, at-home services.

The large transcription services are swallowing up smaller services and hospital accounts voraciously. This is where the bulk of the medical transcription work is these days. I mentioned in an earlier chapter that telecommunication (the ability to send computerized information via telephone) allows transcription services to do work originating in any part of the country.

As an employee of such a service, you will likely be paid according to production rather than hourly—or perhaps it may be a combination of the two. You will be paid so many cents per line of text produced—although what constitutes a line of text is far from standard. (The AAMT recommends payment per character, but most employers are not picking up on it yet.) You may receive insurance benefits, and be paid sick and vacation time, although these latter are sometimes minimal.

Small and one-person services are surviving and thriving, however. They can offer convenience and personalized service—and sometimes quality—that the big guys can't. I know of many such services (run by medical transcriptionists with good business skills) which are doing very well, thank you.

Telecommuting

You may "telecommute," i.e., work from home as an employee. You'll need a computer with a modem. The employer may provide a special receiver that you can plug your headset into for 40 (or 20 or whatever) hours per week, with all the

Work at home as an employee
– ♦ –

work provided for you. And then switch off and take care of your own life. Some people like to work at home like this without the responsibilities and hassles of a home business. More and more employers are doing this, but if they have an on-site facility as well, you may be required to work there for a time first.

Investigate the Work Site

Wherever you choose to work, check it out carefully before hiring on. Just like you're checking out the career right now. Ask about the benefits package, not just how much they pay per line. Visit the site. Do the transcriptionists look happy or harried? Are they helping each other with a difficult word? Do they have time to speak to you and tell you how much they enjoy working there? If you're applying to work as a telecommuter, speak to some of the other telecommuting employees, so you can get the real scoop.

Is the employer concerned about quality—in the transcription work and in the work environment? I've heard some workplaces described as sweatshops. How can we expect others to treat us as skilled professionals if we allow ourselves to be treated like battery hens—where quantity is more important than quality? Beware the employer who asks if you can type 90 words per minute but doesn't care what you type at that speed.

Sweat-
shops

– ♦ –

Rates of Pay

These vary considerably. Not much more than minimum wage in some cases. $50,000 or more per year, in others. Here is a summary:

By The Hour

In rural parts of the country, or in a small office setting, transcriptionists may be paid $6 or $7 an hour. In the big city, in a big hospital, transcriptionists with seniority may be paid $16 to $18 per hour. These figures may be increased by shift differentials (round-the-clock shifts are common in this business), weekend differentials, seniority pay, and production bonuses (extra pay for transcribing more than a set number of lines per shift).

Don't forget the most important thing of all—benefits. Medical insurance, sick pay, vacation pay, and retirement plans are valuable these days. The medical benefits from a medical employer are often very generous. I still work part-time as a medical transcriptionist for a large health maintenance organization, which provides very low-cost medical care and medications for my family. That's worth a lot.

Benefits
– ◆ –

Always factor in the benefits when considering rates of pay.

By The Line

Some employers pay simply on production. Between 5 and 8 cents per line of printed text is the average at the time of writing this book. How many lines will you produce in an eight-hour shift? Until recently, the average was about 1100-1300 lines. With recent improvements in equipment and technology, most medical transcriptionists can comfortably produce 1500 lines per eight hours, and often a lot more. Sometimes there will be a basic hourly rate combined with a per-line rate. Sometimes there will be a benefits package.

Upward Mobility

Some transcription services are large national corporations

with a lot of room for advancement. You may advance to proofreader/editor/quality assurance person. You may become a supervisor or manager of a medical transcription department.

Some employers pay more to CMTs. (see Chapter 7)

You might eventually decide to get into education, sharing the skills you've learned over the years with intelligent adults eager to learn from you. It's something I personally find very satisfying. There's a great need for good medical transcription instructors.

Share your skills
_ ♦ _

You As Contractor

If you're in business for yourself, how much do you charge? 10 to 18 cents per line is the approximate range, depending on where you live and how good you are. This may sound good multiplied by 2,000 lines per eight hours, but there are a lot of expenses to cover.

Still, this is where the big bucks are being made. A good number of my former students already are running busy and successful home-based transcription services. When things get busy, you can hire subcontractors or employees to help you. That's how successful transcription services start. But it takes time and hard work.

Big bucks
_ ♦ _

See Chapter 8 for more about a home transcription business.

7

How do you Become a Medical Transcriptionist?

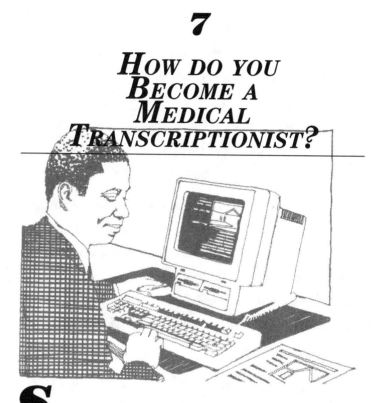

So, you've thought about it carefully and decided this is the career for you. Where do you get your education? The different options are discussed in this chapter.

Occasionally I have a hard time persuading would-be MTs that the medical terminology class they took, their high typing speed, and their fancy new computer are not enough to start them in a medical transcription career.

Your education is going to take *time*. The medical transcriptionist's skills come only from hard work and a lot of practice.

How Long Does It Take?

This is an impossible question to answer. It's like asking how long is a piece of string. It depends on many factors: your past education, your work experience, the amount of time you are able to dedicate to classes, whether or not you're a "word nerd," how quick a learner you are, the quality of your medical transcription education, etc.

There is no set length of time, no standard curriculum after which you are "ready." The employer doesn't care about your Ph.D.in human anatomy, or your certificate of completion from Joe's Quik 'n' Eazy Medical Transcription School. The employer simply wants to know, "Can you do medical transcription?" And you'll have to put on the headphones and show that you can.

If you must have a ballpark figure, it may take 12 to 24 months of education to become "job-ready," to reach the stage where an employer will find you useful. Even then, you'll discover there's so much more to learn. As I've said before, medical transcriptionists, no matter how experienced, are always learning.

Where To Get Your Education

Your choices

– ◆ –

Basically there are three educational routes to becoming a medical transcriptionist: a state-funded community college, a private college, or a private correspondence course. Which is best? If you're lucky enough to live in an area where you have access to all three, and all are of an equally high standard, then I would recommend the first of the three. But there are many factors to consider in this very important decision, and only you can decide what suits you best. Here are some pros and cons for each:

Community Colleges

Pros:

- Cheapest.

- And because they're cheaper, you can afford to spend the length of time that this education really requires.

- Especially suitable if you have a family and full-time job and can only go to school part-time or evenings.

Cons:

- Only two or three starting dates per year.

- Classes tend to fill quickly.

- Long lines on registration day (although some colleges do this by phone now).

Private Colleges

Pros:

- Some colleges have more up-to-date equipment.

- More class hours per week; more condensed course.

- Classes may be smaller.

- More starting dates. Classes often open-ended.

Cons:

- Expensive.

- Many colleges try to cram this education into an impossibly short time. Ask former graduates and employers whether this college gets students job-ready.

- Too many "grant grabbers" and "diploma mills" in the private college business.

Correspondence Course

Pros:

- Less expensive than a private college

- Work at your own pace—at your own place

- No commute

- Ideal if you live in a rural area

Cons:

- More expensive than a community college

The modem ate my homework
– ◆ –

- Although the instructor is usually accessible via an 800 number, there is a definite advantage to classroom interaction with a live instructor and fellow students. Cross your fingers that your valuable work doesn't get lost in the mail or mangled by your modem.

• You need to supply your own computer and transcriber.

• Do you have the discipline to study on your own? Are you undistractible? (kids, phone, TV, fridge) Many of us are less productive without deadlines and structure.

I should say here that of all the correspondence courses out there—and there are many—there are only two or three of them that I have any respect for; and they *are* good. (No, I'm not naming names. This is an independent book. No advertising here.) Yes, many correspondence courses have great advertising, beautiful pages on the Internet, and dynamic free seminars. But most of them are expensive and inadequate. I hope you will do some homework before you spend any money. (See Caveat Emptor below.)

Where are the Schools in my Area?

The AAMT head office (see Further Resources later in this book) will put you in touch with some contact people at your nearest AAMT chapter. This way you can start networking and getting good information about local schools from medical transcriptionists and employers in your community.

Then speak to the instructors (not counselors, not salespeople). They're always happy to answer all your questions. (If they aren't happy to do so, you probably don't want them to teach you.) This is an important first step on the road to becoming a medical transcriptionist. Research carefully.

What Should I Be Looking For?

Your instructor should be (or have been) a medical transcriptionist. It's amazing how many courses are taught by people who've never been medical transcriptionists! Your instructor should be knowledgeable, experienced, enthusiastic, informative, and supportive.

Is the course comprehensive and realistic? Check the class guidelines below. Is there plenty of medical terminology, anatomy, physiology, emphasis on English language, plenty of transcription lab time, a work study program? Few schools score well in every aspect.

Is the course of a realistic length? Rare is the transcription student who's become employed after six to eight months of training—no matter what skills or experience he came in with. Remember, good medical transcriptionists are in demand because this work is hard to do, and takes time to learn.

Should I Learn One Medical Specialty At A Time?

No. Medical transcription schools teach the full medical spectrum. Anything can crop up in any report, and the medical transcriptionist needs to know it all. The head bone's connected to the neck bone, etc. Neurological problems cause orthopedic problems cause psychiatric problems, etc. Once you have your full-spectrum training, you may wish then to choose a particular specialty and become an expert in that. But you'll always need a broad basis of medical knowledge.

Caveat Emptor

Many of us in this profession are tired of the claims made by some colleges and correspondence course sellers that—with a short training course—anyone can "type for doctors." Free literature and free seminars (free to get in, expensive to leave) offer pie in the sky. A dynamic salesperson (not a medical transcriptionist) gives a glowing presentation. She will not mention that most people could never do this work; she'll take anybody's money. She will not mention any of the prerequisite skills you need to have (see Chapter 3). She will not mention that so many students who survive their course feel inadequately trained, with employers turning them away. She will not mention any of the challenges or difficulties of medical transcription (see Chapter 5).

Pie in the sky
– ♦ –

Where does all the money for this expensive advertising and promotion come from? Sucker City, I imagine.

Accreditation of Schools

The AAMT is considering this, and it can't come too soon. The AAMT would "accredit" (approve) schools that offer a realistic medical transcription education conforming to certain criteria. I pray for the day when the general public interested in this profession can get a list of accredited schools and know that they're investing their time and money in a quality education that will get them job-ready.

CMT

Be aware that the only certificate of any real value on your résumé is the CMT (Certified Medical Transcriptionist). This is not offered by any school or government body. It is offered only by our professional association, the American Association for Medical Transcription (AAMT).

What is a certificate?
– ◆ –

Schools and correspondence courses may offer "certificates." These are not CMT certificates and will usually mean very little to an employer because they are offered by all kinds of college for all kinds of reasons.

A good education—particularly through a reputable comprehensive medical transcription course—on your résumé will certainly carry some weight, but it doesn't mean that you are a competent medical transcriptionist. Having the CMT, however, is proof-positive that you are a good medical transcriptionist.

CMT certification is considered to be "entry-level." It's not an easy exam, but a graduate who has worked hard and earned good grades in a comprehensive course ought to be able to pass it. Some prefer to get a year or two of work experience first. The exam is given in two parts. The first is written. Actually, you type your answers into a computer at a special test center. (Centers are located all over the country.) The questions are on English language, grammar, and punctuation, medical terminology, pharmacology, medical records ethics, anatomy, physiology.

You need to pass the first part of the exam in order to take the second, which is a tape of actual medical dictation for transcription. The taped dictation is very fair, but challenging, and a good measure of your abilities. You are allowed very few errors.

When you feel you might be ready to take the CMT exam, ask AAMT to send you a free sample test, so you can see how well you do. This is worthwhile because it costs $150 to take each part of the actual test. However, this small investment in the CMT will reap financial and professional dividends for the rest of your career. You'll get better jobs, better-paying jobs, and move up the ladder more quickly. You'll have more self-respect, and will gain more respect from others. You'll have the proof that you're a true professional.

A profitable investment
— ♦ —

What Classes Shall I Take?

It's important to differentiate whether you want to take a degree course (perhaps an associate's degree as a medical transcription specialist), or whether you simply want to take

Do I need a degree?
— ♦ —

the classes necessary to get you job-ready. A degree may be important to your life goals, but it will probably make little difference to the medical transcription employer.

Since we do not yet have accreditation of medical transcription courses, there is no standard curriculum. No two schools are alike.

Following is a list of the introductory classes that will prepare you for your first medical transcription class.

Medical Terminology

For obvious reasons, this is a standard part of any medical transcription course. It's your introduction to medical language, without which you won't have a clue what the doctors are talking about. The class should be intensive and comprehensive. No "quickies" here. Some students want to bypass the medical terminology class, saying they worked as a nurse or an insurance biller or in some other medical profession. It is important to realize that the medical transcriptionist—or medical language specialist—needs medical language skills far beyond those of virtually everyone else in medicine. (Many medical professionals use these words, but not so many know how to spell them correctly.)

Business English/Fundamentals of English

Without advanced language skills, we cannot understand,

interpret, and accurately document some of the very unfamiliar, ungrammatical, unusual, and erroneous dictation that will come our way. Unless you have a degree in English, or are an experienced writer, don't doubt the importance of an English class. High school standard isn't very high these days. Poor language skills are the commonest problem in our transcription classes. Don't be overconfident about your abilities here.

Word Processing

Just minimal requirements here. Take a basic word processing class if you've never used a word processor before. It needn't be comprehensive or a semester long. A basic one-day class would be ample. You don't need to know complex word processing functions. WordPerfect and Microsoft Word happen to be the most widely used, but they're not necessarily the best or the ones you prefer to use. When you know the basics of one word processing program, you'll find the others remarkably similar and easy to learn.

Typing

Again, just minimal requirements. If you don't have 40 words per minute, take a typing speed class at the start of your medical transcription training. After this, typing speed should not be an issue until the end of your training. It will automatically increase with all of your transcription practice. If you haven't reached 65 wpm as you near graduation, then is the time to take a typing speed class. Don't worry about speed until then. Concentrate on *content*. When you have accurate content, *then* you can speed it up.

And Then Your First Medical Transcription Class

When you have some basic skills in the above subjects, then you can begin to use them in your first Medical Transcription class, where you'll learn the art of putting medical reports together from dictation. You'll learn the different types of report, the styles, abbreviations, and technical jargon used. You'll encounter the constant grammatical questions that can make sense or nonsense of the reports. You'll develop a keen ear and a detective's mind. You'll encounter more and more difficult dictation, and medical terms and procedures you've never heard of. You'll learn a whole lot about medicine. Usually at least one Advanced Medical Transcription class will follow.

Putting it all together
– ♦ –

Anatomy/Physiology/Pathophysiology/ Advanced Medical Terminology

Take as many of these classes as you can concurrent to your medical transcription classes. The more you know about medicine, the sooner you'll be a medical transcriptionist.

Work Experience

This might be your most valuable class. Not every college offers it, but it's a definite plus if you can find it. You'll get college credits and guidance while working in a real work setting—surely the best education you can get. And sometimes even job offers result, although you should not expect this to happen as a rule.

Placement Service

Be warned that if a private college or correspondence course advertises a "placement" service, this may be with just one company (sometimes a subsidiary of the college) with some long-term contract for cheap labor. Find out more about the "placement." Speak to former graduates.

How to Get Your First Job

Your instructor and your local AAMT network will be your best resources when you're ready to look for work.

In Chapter 5, I mentioned that getting your first job can seem like a difficult hurdle to cross. But I've never seen a capable student who did not cross it.

The best advice I can give is to study hard and get involved.

During your school time, practice as much as you can. Take

**Immerse
yourself**

– ♦ –

all the related classes you can. Read all the medical material

you can. Browse through your medical dictionary and Gray's

Anatomy whenever you have a chance. Look things up. Learn

meanings of words, not just spellings. Understand how they

fit into context. You'll learn tons more on the job, but an

employer wants to hire someone with a strong foundation of

medical knowledge.

Get involved. Network with your fellow medical transcrip-

tionists (and employers, and fellow students) at AAMT

Network

– ♦ –

meetings (see Chapter 9), the on-line forums (see Further

Resources), and with your instructor and fellow students in

the classroom. These people will give you the support and

confidence you need to go out there—knowing you're a well-

trained professional worthy of employment in this field.

**The
personal
touch**

– ♦ –

I always recommend the personal touch when job-seek-

ing—actually visiting a transcription department and its

people. You'll make much more of an impression that way,

even if they do politely decline your services. Your enthusi-

asm and professional look may be remembered next time

there's a vacant position. Especially if you follow up with a

phone call every month or two afterwards. Whereas a résumé

sent to the Personnel Department is just another piece of

paper filed away with thousands more.

How I Got My First Job in Medical Transcription

I've never been particularly outgoing, but when I was just out of vocational school, I had the confidence to visit all the local hospital transcription departments, just to see what they were like, and to see if there were any vacancies. Most of the supervisors or transcriptionists found time to talk with me. Eventually I talked with a transcription supervisor who was desperate for a clerk in the transcription department. She said I could practice transcribing tapes anytime my work was caught up. I took the clerical job and made sure my work was always caught up. I took every opportunity to transcribe tapes and gain valuable experience. A few months later when a transcriptionist position opened up, I got the job.

Bottom line: Get a good education, train hard, then be prepared to advertise your skills. The work is out there waiting for you.

8

Your Home Medical Transcription Business

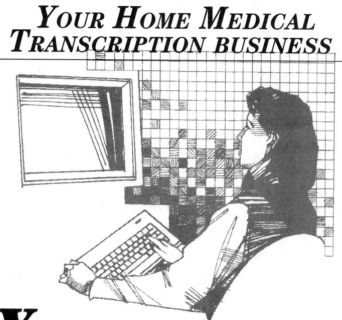

You've seen all the ads and articles and magazines touting the glamor of home business. It sounds great, doesn't it? No boss. No commute. Work when you want. Take off when you want. Tax benefits. Independence. Freedom.

Millions of dollars are being made in home business today. Or should I say, in selling the *dream* of home business. Hold onto your credit cards. Speak to people who *have* a home business and get a solid dose of reality. Your local library and the Small Business Administration will have some good, honest material on what it really takes to run a home business.

Hold onto your credit cards
– ♦ –

It's important to emphasize that you will need to success-fully accomplish Step 1—become a good medical transcrip-tionist—before you tackle Step 2—start a home medical transcription business. Step 1 needs all your time and energy, so first things first. Have patience (one of the virtues of a successful medical transcriptionist).

You'll need one to two years of education (see Chapter 7) and at least a year of actual work experience before it's realistic to start a successful home medical transcription business. Yes, there's plenty of work out there, but it's competitive and you'll have to be good at what you do. Success and money—in any business—don't just fall out of the sky. They come to those who train hard, work hard, and pay their dues.

Keep out of the danger zone

— ♦ —

When you do reach Step 2, and are ready to start your business, you will need to be well prepared. Home businesses have an amazingly high failure rate, and if you think you can start one without serious research (from the experts, not salespeople), then you're heading for the danger zone.

This chapter does not go through all the nuts and bolts of setting up a home business. Bookstores and libraries are full of such books.

This chapter does contain a rundown of the equipment you'll find in the medical transcriptionist's home office. I do this reluctantly, because technology changes so fast; my list may be obsolete by the time you read this book. It will certainly be pretty out of date by the time you're in a position to start your business. But I yield to popular demand!

What is important—and what I will address primarily in this chapter—is that you consider *every single aspect* of a home-based medical transcription business, and whether it's right for you. After all, a lot of medical transcriptionists are much happier *without* the responsibilities of a business. They would rather work for someone else (whether at home or at a worksite) and feel as free as a bird the other 16 hours per day.

Home-Based Medical Transcription—A Trend of the Future

There is a definite trend toward home-based medical transcription. Employers' offices and work sites cost money. No need to pay for them if the work can be done in someone's home. And with modern telecommunications technology, it can.

Once you've spent some time with a hospital or large transcription service and proved your skill and reliability, they may fix you up to continue as an employee from your home.

Some national transcription companies employ *only* home-based medical transcriptionists.

Alternatively, you can be a self-employed independent contractor, with a computer, a modem, and a telephone line, working for doctors around the country from your mountain cabin in Vermont or your beachside villa in Hawaii.

So When Can I Start?

There's nothing to stop you from going straight from school and starting your home business—if you can convince the doctors you can do it. Some of my students have done it, and a few have even succeeded. But by starting too early, it will actually take you *longer* to reach success. You're going to feel very inexperienced. You'll be learning on the job. Without a teacher. Learning when you should be earning. Working at a speed that brings you minimum wage, if you're lucky. Prone to making mistakes and losing accounts. Getting frustrated. This is the slow way. You'll never be a top-notch medical transcriptionist at this rate.

Wait!
– ♦ –

It would be smarter to stuff as much learning as you can into an intensive 12-24-month medical transcription education program, with all of the expert advice, facilities and structure available there. Then expand on that education in an employment setting for a year or two, where you can build a firm foundation of medical transcription knowledge. Doing it this way, you'll be far more advanced—say three years from today—than if you had spent a year or less in school and had learned only from the work of one or two doctor clients in your home business. With more intensive training and work experience under your belt, you'll be ready to tackle the demands of a home-based medical transcription business. You'll be able to handle *any* work that comes along. Any doctor. Any medical terms. Any specialty. Able to compete for *all* that transcription work out there. Ready to get your CMT. You'll be competent, confident, and capable. And making money.

Most medical transcriptionists will recommend the same.

How Much Can I Make?

There are a few medical transcriptionists who make a lot of money in this business. An independent contractor, working hard, can make $50,000 or more per year. Consolidate your skills for a few years. Continue your medical education. Develop good business practices. Earn a reputation for quality and service. Get more work than you can handle. Hire a few subcontractors. The sky's the limit.

Is it Expensive to Start up?

In today's world of expensive high technology, medical transcription departments and services can spend many thousands of dollars on hardware, software, and reference

Expensive Toys
– ♦ –

materials. My advice, though, to the new business start-up is to buy the expensive toys when your business succeeds, because you can do well enough at first without most of them.

I started a successful home medical transcription business in 1983 with an electronic typewriter, a used transcriber (the desktop tape player), and three second-hand reference books. But the most important tools I had were the knowledge, experience, skill, and reputation for quality that I had developed in my five years as a hospital medical transcriptionist. It was because of these tools that I immediately gained my first contract—overload transcription from the largest hospital in San Diego. I picked up other contracts just as easily, and sometimes wished I had four heads and eight hands to do all the work that was available to me.

No, you don't need to spend a lot of money to start a home medical transcription service. But you do need to be a good medical transcriptionist.

You'll learn about the latest and greatest new equipment during your schooling and through your AAMT network and professional journals. Digital recording, speech-recognition software, high-speed modems have appeared from nowhere in the last year or two. There is software that can almost guess what you're going to type. Medical reference books are built into our spellcheckers. Etc., etc.

What Equipment Will I Need?

As of the writing of this book, this is the equipment you'll find in a home-based medical transcription office:

A computer with a word processing program. The most basic word processing program does perfectly well for the medical transcriptionist. We don't need the magical features performed by the expensive, big-name word processing programs. Remember, we did this work on typewriters not so long ago! As your business succeeds, you may find that an investment in one of the more sophisticated word processing programs allows you to work with more time-saving software. Decide whether it's worth it when you reach that stage.

By the way, if you haven't a computer now, this is one item you might consider purchasing early in your training, once you've decided you love medical transcription. Any extra practice you can do outside of the classroom will get you job-ready all the sooner. A good school will have a computer lab available to you for this purpose; but if you have the budget, your own computer is a good investment in your future.

What to look for in a computer purchase: You don't need the latest and greatest with all the bells and whistles. (Your kids and spouse will take it over if you get one of those.) Never mind the bits and bytes and megahertz and milliseconds that the computer journals ramble on about. They're of little importance to medical transcriptionists. Keyboard and screen (or monitor) are your priorities.

Some computer *keyboards* are poor for medical transcriptionists. They're badly laid out, or don't have a receptive
touch. (Think carpal tunnel syndrome.) The most important
thing you can do when purchasing a computer is to give the
keyboard a good workout. (Tell the salesperson why you're
rapidly typing on a keyboard that isn't even hooked up to a
computer!) Some keyboards have small "return/enter" and
"backspace" keys. That's not important to the 95% of computer users who "peck" rather than type. But it's important
that these be larger-size keys for those of us with flying
fingers and making 100,000 keystrokes a day. (I counted 'em!)

If you're going to gaze at a *computer screen* for eight hours
a day, you'd be wise to "eye-test" a few before making your
purchase. Makes sure it has a "dot pitch" of 0.28 or lower.

A good-quality *printer* is important once you're a professional medical transcriptionist. Inkjet printers are finally
reaching acceptable print quality, but laser print looks so
much better and will really help you sell the image of quality
to your clients. Excellent laser printers are now very affordable. Although inkjet printers are cheaper than laser printers,
you'll spend more in the long run for replacement ink car-
tridges.

Cassette tapes will be around for a year or two yet, but by the
time you're ready to start your home business, *digital record-
ing/playback systems* will be the standard. Digital systems are
already used by hospital transcription departments and the

larger transcription services. These systems come in the form of a little box of technology that connects to your computer and your telephone. Sometimes it will have a separate monitor showing information about the dictation; sometimes your existing computer monitor does that job. Some digital systems are simply circuit boards installed inside your computer! Hooked up to your telephone line, this system enables your clients to call in and dictate their reports.

There's still a lot of dictation done onto cassette tapes. Microcassettes may be a little more widely used than standard cassettes, but most self-employed medical transcriptionists have transcribers for both.

The *transcriber* is the desktop tape player with a footpedal control that frees your hands for keyboard work. These machines are surprisingly expensive (anywhere from $200 to $600), but used machines are plentiful as more offices convert to digital systems. Get the standard-size transcriber first, because educational tapes come in that size. A used transcriber is another useful early purchase for the medical transcription student, to give you that extra practice at home. Look in the classifieds for office auctions; or in the yellow pages for office supply stores that refurbish used equipment; or ask around at your local AAMT chapter meeting (see Chapter 9).

The *headsets* supplied with transcribers are often of low quality. A few dollars well spent here will make your work a lot easier. I've always used a set of hi-fi stereo headphones, light-weight, comfortable, great quality, and not much more expensive than the cheap, ear-hurting plastic supplied by the transcriber makers. A stereo-to-mono adapter pin is cheap and available at any electronics store. Headphones of this quality will let you distinctly hear every word of Dr. Mushmouth. He'll sound just like Luciano Pavarotti! Well, almost.

Be ergono-mically aware

— ♦ —

In an earlier chapter I said that a major difficulty in this work is sitting at a computer for eight hours a day. It may be impossible unless you have the right chair. While there are many office furnishings that will make your work more comfortable (the right desk, good lighting, etc.), your *chair* is the most important piece of furniture and should be near the top of your list of priority equipment. Try out some chairs at your local office supply store that are designed specifically for the eight-hour-a-day keyboard person. The right chair will swivel, have five feet set on wheels, and be adjustable up and down, and forward and back. It will give you comfort; and more than any other "tool of your trade," it will increase your productivity.

Reference books are also important tools and can drain your bank account very quickly. Again, you can start very cheaply and build your collection as you build your business. A used medical dictionary (Dorland's and Stedman's are the medical transcriptionists' favorites) can be acquired cheaply from someone at your AAMT meeting who just bought a new one. A PDR (Physicians' Desk Reference) may be available free from your local pharmacist or family physician when they've just received the latest annual edition. Beyond those, there are helpful reference books that list medical terms according to specialty, books with just surgical terms, abbreviations, phonetic spellings, and many more. You'll meet them in your classroom. And don't forget two essential reference books: a good English dictionary, and the telephone directory.

Many of these medical reference books are being converted into *software* for easier access via your computer. Other popular software is the "macro" program, where common words, phrases, sentences, or paragraphs can be brought into your document with a couple of keystrokes. Spellcheckers, despite their limitations, can be helpful for a final proofread of your work.

If you haven't a *modem* already, you'll certainly need one as a home-based medical transcriptionist. In the years to come, we'll be doing less collecting and delivering of cassette tapes, and more transferring of our work via modem.

A *fax machine* and *photocopy machine* are not essential to start with, but well worth having as your business grows. They're becoming quite affordable.

I think these are the basics. Read your *professional journals* (see Further Resources at the back of this book) to keep up with the latest advances and to see ads for the newest toys.

This will never change — ♦ —   The technology we use changes every day. But one thing will remain constant: the combined knowledge of medicine and language that only a medical language specialist/medical transcriptionist possesses and is able to process at lightning speed using the current technology.

Take care of your education. Your other tools are incidental.

* * *

The Pros and Cons of a Home-Based Medical Transcription Business

Pros

No more treadmill — ♦ —   *Freedom/independence/flexible hours* — You don't have to work 9 to 5 for the rest of your life. Or the graveyard shift. Or have only Saturdays and Sundays off, when the stores and even the parks are crowded. You don't have to feel like a mouse inside one of those ever-spinning wheels, going nowhere. You can make your own life. Get back in control. Set your own hours.

Yes, it takes time and hard work to get there. But a lot of people are there. Why not you? Did you know that people running successful home businesses average far more than 40 hours of work per week? And they love every minute of it.

Of course, when Dr. Procrastinator calls at 8:00 p.m. Sunday evening—just as you were settling down with your family to watch a movie—with some dictation she needs by tomorrow morning, you'll realize there are just a few limitations to your freedom and flexibility You don't want to lose that contract, do you?

No commute — Yay! No argument with this one. Time is precious. We have better things to do with our lives than sit on the freeway. What could we do with the hour or two we save each day? Make more money. Play. Relax. I can think of a hundred things.

A bonus of time

– ♦ –

Save money on office clothes — Work in your jammies if you want. Remember, though, that you'll need to look and feel professional when you're out on business, meeting clients. Many home-based workers like to wear professional clothes even when they're working at home. It helps put them in an "at work" mode and thus be more productive. It gives the "at work" message to your family too.

Best boss in the world — Work for #1! But don't be *too* nice to yourself. (See below under *How's your self-discipline* and *Be a darn good manager*)

Be closer to your kids — Minor advantage here. Don't expect to do this work with children running around your feet.

Certainly your children can be nearby and you can be available for them at short notice. But they need to be in another room in a supervised setting, aware that Mommy or Daddy is "at work." Childcare and medical transcription do not mix. Medical transcription is intensive work that requires your utmost attention and concentration.

Cons

Taxes — First of all, they're complicated. Second, you've got to do them yourself, or pay someone else to do them. Certainly you'll have to spend time on detailed record keeping. Thirdly, you pay more. And you'll need a business license, perhaps a fictitious business name filing fee, zoning permit.... It amazes me to hear how many people think home business people have a good thing going with taxes and can deduct anything and everything. Any home business person will tell you that's not the case. The IRS and the Government are not kind to the self-employed. Let's get onto the next topic before I feel sick.

No benefits — The medical benefits, pension plans, vacation pay, sick pay we all took for granted as an employee are gone. Take a vacation or get sick? Hope you made enough money the rest of the year to cover it. Health insurance is available for the self-employed, but it's not cheap. Start your own pension plan with an IRA or Keogh. Lobby your Congress people to enact better tax incentives and health insurance for the self-employed. Join a home business organization for information and support.

Cyclical work — It's hard to maintain the ideal balance of work. Usually there's too much or too little. When Dr. Windbag goes on vacation, there's a hole in your bank account. Or *you* want to take a vacation. Will Dr. Windbag find someone else to do her transcription while you're gone? And will you get that work back when you return? Perhaps Dr. Windbag's clientele grows, and thus the volume of transcription she loads on you. Then her partner sees how good your work is and would like you to do his transcription too. You don't want to turn down work, but suddenly you're overwhelmed. It can be feast or famine for the home-based medical transcriptionist (and feast is by far the more common).

**feast or
famine**

— ♦ —

Networking with your fellow self-employed medical transcriptionists through the AAMT will help you balance your workload in situations like these, but it can be a bit of a rollercoaster.

Cabin fever — It was mentioned in an earlier chapter that a medical transcriptionist has to have an independent streak. It applies even more to the medical transcriptionist working at home. If you're the gregarious sort, or the restless sort who needs to get out and smell the roses, or the traffic fumes, then this solitary workplace may not suit you.

Cost of equipment and materials — As I've said, you can get started very cheaply. But when you see all the time-saving toys out there, you won't be able to resist buying some, particularly if they enhance your productivity (= income). Don't forget the cost of service contracts and repairs. "Down time" can be very expensive.

Competition — There are others out there hustling after the same work you are. You'll have to be better than they are. Market yourself. Continue your education. Go that extra mile.

What Skills Do I Need To Succeed In A Home-Based Medical Transcription Business?

Be a darn good medical transcriptionist

Get a lot of experience first by working for someone else. That way, you'll be ready for anything that comes your way— unusual terms, new drugs, poor dictation, lousy recording quality. Because now you'll be on your own. You need to keep that contract. You're being paid by production, so you need to *produce*.

Be a darn good marketer

It's no use being a darn good medical transcriptionist if no one but you knows it. You will need to spend time on marketing your services. There are good books on this subject in your library and bookstore. It's a very important aspect of your work. It's competitive out there, and customers can disappear quick as a wink. *Present yourself* like a professional. *Feel* like a professional. *Be* a professional.

Be a darn good manager

Transcription, marketing, paperwork, accounting, equipment maintenance, billing, and a few hundred other things all need to be organized and taken care of by the business owner—you! Oh, and you probably have a family to fit in there somewhere too. You may never have been a manager before. You may have subcontractors or employees to manage. It's not easy. Again, there are good small-business management resources available at your library and through the Small Business Administration.

Busy busy busy
– ◆ –

How's Your Self-Discipline?

No taking breaks to watch the soaps or the football game. No long phone calls to friends. No playing with the kids. Not during work time anyway. You chose a home business for flexible hours. But once you've set your hours for the day, stick to them rigidly. If your work schedule for today is 9:30 a.m. to 1:30 p.m., then 8:00 p.m. to midnight, remind your family, and yourself, that you're at work during those hours and not to be interrupted except in an emergency. Lose that structure, lose your business.

No soaps
– ◆ –

Continuing Education

You'll need to invest some time and money in continuing education. You might call it "sharpening your tools." You need to keep up with the many developments in medicine. This is available through the AAMT (see Chapter 9) and most medical facilities.

Get your CMT

By attaining CMT standard, you know you've taken yourself to a professional level. Potential clients will know that too. Anyone can call herself a medical transcriptionist, but not just anyone can call herself a Certified Medical Transcriptionist.

Summary

A home-based medical transcription business is a full-time occupation. A dedication. A responsibility. And for someone who works hard and has the right skills and attributes, it can be very rewarding.

9

The AAMT and Professionalism

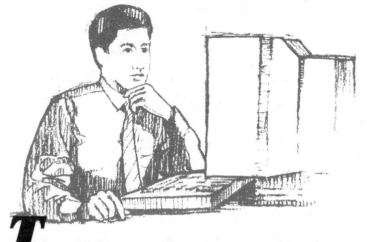

*T*here are few jobs that require this much skill and pay so modestly. Although our work requires essentially the same skills as those of court reporters and medical writers—who are better paid than medical transcriptionists—we have, until recently, allowed ourselves to be categorized (and paid) as clerical workers. Many employers' job descriptions continue to classify medical transcriptionists along the lines of "typists with a medical dictionary!"

In 1978, an enthusiastic group of medical transcriptionists, recognizing this disparity, formed the American Association for Medical Transcription. Now we are 10,000 strong. 100,000 would be stronger (there are at least that number of medical transcriptionists). We're working on it.

Strength in numbers
— ♦ —

The AAMT is our professional association. Independent. Nonprofit. The AAMT is our representative in high places—with the government, with the AMA, and with other professional organizations. It provides business conferences, educators conferences, conventions, student workshops, medical lectures, and meetings for members on a national, state, and local level—a hundred different ways of networking, coordinating, learning, sharing information, and growing. The AAMT is our network. It is us—the MTs who know that collectively we can move mountains!

Our voice
– ◆ –

What's in it for me?

Money! Well no, they won't send you a check every year. You'll have to send one to them. But the AAMT member is an *informed* medical transcriptionist, knows where the jobs are, knows about the latest developments in the field, in medicine, in technology, knows all about the money-saving software and hardware, gets the latest information on running a business, etc., etc. At local chapter meetings, you'll be networking with fellow MTs, students, instructors, and employers. Because of all this, I'll wager that the average AAMT member MT is better paid than the average nonmember MT. So there *is* money in it for you.

The rewards
– ◆ –

All professionals have professional associations, and AAMT dues are cheaper than most, with discount rates for students.

The cost of tools and equipment is part of every professional's life. Our most important tools are medical knowledge and information. As supplied by the AAMT, these tools are a bargain and a profitable investment.

Being a part of the AAMT makes you feel more like a professional. You'll realize more of your potential. Professionally, I have grown by leaps and bounds as an AAMT member.

AAMT offers professional certification via the CMT (see Chapter 7), and some of the continuing education required to maintain that certification.

AAMT will help you keep up with the rapid changes going on in the industry.

AAMT offers comradeship and support. When you're self-employed and too much or too little work is coming in, where are you going to to find someone to help out? At your local AAMT meetings, of course.

AAMT offers education. Most chapters offer monthly meetings where medical professionals give informative presentations on the latest medical procedures. The medical knowledge we gain is one of the major "tools of our trade."

Support
– ♦ –

AAMT meetings help students gain confidence and meet fellow students, employers, and more experienced transcriptionists. More and more chapters are holding special "student day" workshops to support those who are the future of our profession.

What's in it for all of us?

Medical transcription is a profession in flux. Major changes are going on. There is great potential for medical transcriptionists to gain more autonomy and appreciation for what they do. But it won't happen without their (your) active participation. Don't let anyone call us "transcribers" (the machines that play tapes). Don't let anyone call us "typists." Don't let anyone tell us that "anyone can do this job; you don't need more than a few months of training; you don't need professional certification."

I hope that some of you will eventually become "activists" in the organization. It's great to see so many of my former and current students actively involved in our local chapter. One of them is president-elect! Everyone has something to offer— perhaps as a committee member, a board member, a speaker, a writer, a fund raiser, an educator, a mentor, an

A democracy
— ♦ —

organizer, a voice. You can participate at the local and/or national level. AAMT is a democracy, and all are welcome.

10

Is There a Future in Medical Transcription?

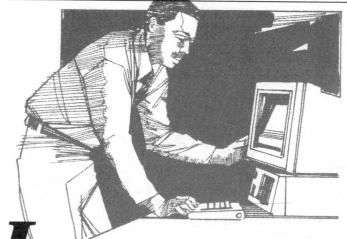

Is there a future in medical transcription? Will there be a glut in the market? Will speech-recognition technology take over?

"Yes"," I don't think so," and "no" are my respective answers.

Medical Transcriptionists Are In Demand

The National Institutes for Health recently predicted a need for 58% more medical transcriptionists by the year 2005. A report from the U.S. Bureau of Labor predicted a need for 51% more medical transcriptionists and medical secretaries in the next few years. Other surveys make similar predictions.

Predictions
— ♦ —

The demand for medical transcriptionists is growing. The population is increasing. And in our litigious society, the trend—and legal requirement—is most definitely towards printed rather than handwritten documentation.

There are few, if any, unemployed medical transcriptionists. There may be some between jobs who have just been laid off because an employer is "downsizing" or "outsourcing" (transferring transcription work to another service). But the work is still there; it's just in the hands of different employers. Once when I was laid off as a hospital employee, I immediately took on that hospital's work as an independent contractor in my home business!

Some new medical transcriptionists, recently graduated, have a hard time getting started because some employers in this field are so reluctant to take on even well-trained apprentices. (See Chapter 5, Getting Your First Job.) Other graduates looking for work, alas, make the awful discovery that their course of training was insufficient. Having read this book and been forewarned, I trust that *you* will not fall into this situation.

Health care is relatively recession proof. We just can't do without it. Whatever changes occur in health care, we will always need accurate patient records. There's a certain amount of security there for the medical transcriptionist.

Will There Be Too Many Medical Transcriptionists?

There is certainly more interest in medical transcription today, more publicity about it, and more training courses available. But not everyone survives the training. Many drop out because they did not realize what they were getting into. Maybe they believed sales pitches and were seduced by the glamor of running a profitable business from home. They didn't realize it required a lot of hard work!

The fact remains that only a special few people can do this kind of work, and the supply seems to be keeping up with the demand.

Supply and demand
– ◆ –

Concerns

I'm not without concerns for the future of our profession. For although the demand for medical transcriptionists will undeniably grow, will that demand be for *quality* medical transcriptionists? Or will the demanders accept lower quality in an effort to cut costs? Doctors expect the best. But increasingly the choices are made for them by cost-conscious managers and administrators who don't know the difference between accurate transcription and transcription with "just a few mistakes in it." And the latter can be done by a far broader spectrum of the population. The managers and administrators may choose to have the work done by

lower-quality, lower-paid medical transcriptionists—
keeping pay rates low for *all* medical transcriptionists.

Certification Would Help

The healthcare industry—and the public—expects its physicians to have medical doctorates, its nurses to be registered,
its radiology technicians to be certified, etc., etc. In any walk
of life, you are safer having services performed by a
credentialed professional.

**Not
enough
CMTs
— ♦ —**

Unfortunately, there is currently no requirement that
medical transcription be done by credentialed medical
transcriptionists. I wish more MTs would obtain certification.
Very few do. They say they can get work without it. Which
may be true today. But how can we expect employers to treat
us and pay us like professionals if we don't treat ourselves as
such? Look at any other profession. They protect themselves
and the integrity of their professions by requiring degrees or
certification in order to practice. If more of us get our CMTs,
then employers are more likely to recognize that this is a
special skill. If only 1 in 10 MTs has a CMT, some cost-
conscious employers may continue to think that this is
unskilled work. There will be a large, mediocre, low-paid
work force to choose from. On the other hand, if 9 in 10 MTs
have a CMT, the employer is more likely to say, "I'm not going
to hire the unqualified one. I'd better hire a CMT."

Some of the "old-timer" medical transcriptionists did fine without certification, but things are changing fast in this field. A lot of newcomers, having trained hard and struggled to get started, realize that their skills and hard work deserve some recognition, and that they deserve some professional security.

I hope that all of you entering this profession will make certification your goal. And be active to ensure that others do the same. I sincerely believe it's the most important thing we can do for the secure future of our profession.

Overseas Transcription Services

Some medical transcriptionists are concerned for the future of our profession in that some U.S. transcription services are having their work done overseas, in countries where English is spoken (e.g., Barbados, Jamaica, India, Ireland). How will this affect the labor market for medical transcriptionists in the U.S.? Labor rates in these countries are much lower. The technology required by a U.S. corporation to set up an overseas facility is relatively cheap and simple, and tax breaks and foreign government subsidies are in their favor. English is very well spoken and taught in many countries around the world, and perhaps even to a higher degree than in the U.S! So training these foreign workers is not difficult or expensive. Good cheap labor to do the work formerly done by U.S. workers.

It seems so far that these overseas operations are in good hands, and that quality assurance is high. If the work they produce is CMT standard, then I have no complaints. I am not a protectionist. If the work is substandard, however, then it's unhealthy for our profession and for U.S. health care that unskilled medical transcriptionists (of any nationality) transcribe our medical reports. I *am* protective of our professional standards.

Speech Recognition Technology

Earlier I mentioned the basic process of medical transcription, where doctors simply pick up a microphone or telephone and dictate the information fresh from memory. Skilled personnel (medical transcriptionists) take care of the rest. Quick and easy for the doctor, who can then continue with *doctor* work. It's for this reason, more than any other, that I do not see speech recognition technology—or any technology—*replacing* medical transcriptionists.

Doctors have better things to do
— ♦ —

Speech Recognition Technology (SRT) takes just too much of the doctor's valuable time—with the initial training, and with the data entry process itself. Most doctors do not have the spelling, punctuation, language skills, or the patience of the medical transcriptionist, and most will be happy to leave this work to us and spend their time doing what they do best—treating patients. Time and money are being wasted when the doctor has to do work that others can do much better and for far less cost.

The complexities of our language are immense, and SRT is a million miles from emulating the human brain. Even a hundred years from now, when the SRT can do a passable job of interpreting doctors' dictation, will we trust the computer's version without any proofreading? No. It's far too dangerous. There will *always* be a need for medical language specialists.

Human beings required
– ♦ –

I wish the reader could hear some medical dictation. Do so if you get a chance. You'll see then how difficult (or impossible) it will be for Speech Recognition Technology to safely handle this kind of work. (See "Great Dictators I Have Known" in Chapter 5.) Dr. X., for example, is the nicest psychiatrist you could ever know. He always wears a beanie cap with a propeller on it at office parties. But his dictation, well, it leaves something to be desired. Especially when he's behind schedule and has a patient waiting. Give that dictation to an SRT computer and it would explode. It's dictated at 120 mph. His own name, the introductory headings, and the first couple of sentences are a mush of sound that bear no resemblance to the actual words intended. Only experience and detective work tell the human transcriptionist what these words are—and which words belong in the report and which do not.

Exploding computers
– ♦ –

How would SRT handle the situations I discussed in Chapter 2 ("So What Goes On Between The Keystrokes")—

the endless permutation of words and phrases that sound the same but can be interpreted in different ways? Should we trust a machine to correctly distinguish between "reduced 2.5 mg" and "reduced to 0.5 mg"?

There *is* room for voice recognition technology in medical transcription, and it is being used already. There are many standard/routine medical reports where everything is basically the same each time except for a few variable details—a few blanks to be filled in. Doctors working with voice recognition computers could handle these reports safely enough. The medical transcriptionist, however, could process this information even more efficiently if the doctor preferred just to rattle it off into a telephone. We have the same kind of "fill-in-the-blank" templates and macros on our computers.

But this is not the work that takes up most of the medical transcriptionist's time and skills. The most voluminous and time-consuming documentation concerns the abnormal/nonroutine cases, where "fill-in-the-blank" reports just don't work.

I see the *medical transcriptionist* using SRT, i.e., redictating the doctor's dictation and monitoring it and tidying it up as it goes onto the screen. This will be an efficient process. It will save a lot of time and keystrokes (and carpal tunnel syndrome!). Some medical transcriptionists are doing this already.

I'll finish this discussion by relating a story I read in Newsweek by one of the editors who was trying out SRT. Every time her neighbor sneezed, the SRT computer would type out "Georgetown."

Atchoo!

— ♦ —

Other New Technologies

The electronic patient record, sometimes known as the computerized patient record, looms in our future. This means that instead of a medical chart full of paper, medical records will take the form of a computerized database. Will this be the end of the medical transcriptionist? Hardly. The information still needs to be entered into the record with the same degree of quality and accuracy. Exactly the same skills are required to transcribe the information onto the computer page as onto the printed page.

Digital Recording is replacing tape recording, although the latter will still be around for a while. Digital recording goes straight onto computer chips. The sound quality is better and the recorded material more accessible. You can instantly go straight from the beginning of Dictation #2 to the end of Dictation #2 to half-way through Dictation #5, etc., just with clicks of a button.

Modems are very useful in medical transcription. First, the digitalized dictation can be sent instantaneously via modem through telephone lines to transcriptionists around the country. Then the transcribed results can be sent back via modem to the hospital or transcription service office and printed out there.

The *stenotype* or shorthand machine, as used by court reporters, is not new technology, but it's relatively new to medical transcription. With this machine, the court reporter can very quickly and efficiently record dictation in the form of shorthand notes. These notes, which once had to be read and typed into regular text, can now be "read" by computer software. Obviously, the court reporter has to carefully monitor and edit that "reading" or "translation" as it comes out on the computer screen, but it certainly saves a lot of time and keyboard work.

Some people thought at first that medical transcriptionists could increase their productivity by anywhere from 50 to 80% using a stenotype machine and the appropriate software. But as we saw in an earlier chapter, medical transcription is a lot more than simply robot-like data entry. Medical transcriptionists with court reporter-level stenotype skills tried it out, but at most could realize a productivity increase of 10 to 15%. Others found little or no increase in productivity.

If you can realize a 10% productivity increase, it's not to be sneezed at, and any medical transcriptionist with stenotype skills would be advised to try to adapt them to medical transcription.

Would it be worthwhile for a medical transcription student to learn stenotype as part of her education? Stenotype is actually very easy to learn. But it's much more difficult to reach the high speeds required for courtroom employability or practical use in medical transcription.

To broaden your career options, you might even consider taking classes in both court reporting and medical transcription. Some colleges offer both, since both subjects have a lot in common—the listening skills, the language skills, the dexterity.

Court reporting
– ♦ –

Time-saving software includes programs that can bring to our screen—with just one or two keystrokes—an outline for the report we're about to transcribe with the patient information and all the report headings already filled in. There are programs that will print out on the screen words like "esophagogastroduodenoscopy" or phrases like, "The patient is a well-developed, well-nourished male," with just one or two keystrokes. There are programs that have sophisticated memories and predict (and type) the next few words for us! (Some careful editing skills required here by the medical transcriptionist.) It's hard to imagine what the software developers will come up with next!

Let's not forget our good old friend the *spellchecker*, which has become quite sophisticated over the last few years. Nowadays spellcheckers contain comprehensive medical dictionaries and more.

But will spellcheckers replace a medical transcriptionist's skills? Hardly.

A spellchecker will catch about 25% of your mistakes. Only the spellchecker in an experienced medical transcriptionist's brain is capable of safely proofreading a medical document. Words can be spelled correctly but be utterly wrong and out of context. The Journal of the AAMT used to regularly publish a medical report in each issue that had been "okayed" by a spellchecker. And it was garbage! Full of mistakes.

An abdomen full of groceries

— ♦ —

Imagine you're an experienced MT, transcribing Dr. Windbag's third gallbladder removal of the day, and part of your brain is thinking about other things. (It does happen.) Suddenly your grocery list appears in the patient's abdomen. The spellchecker wouldn't catch it, as long as you'd spelled your tomatoes and potatoes correctly.

Summary

There are rapid changes going on in technology and in the healthcare environment that affect medical transcription. Yet it remains that there will always be a need for skilled medical transcriptionists/medical language specialists—experts with the English language, wise and up-to-the-minute in their knowledge of medicine, and skilled with the latest technology in order to safely and accurately process and document medicolegal information.

It will take someone special. You?

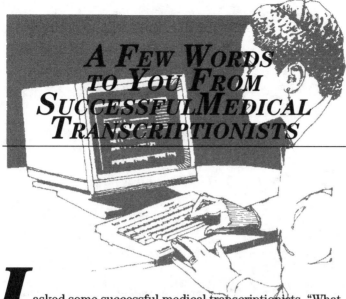

A FEW WORDS TO YOU FROM SUCCESSFUL MEDICAL TRANSCRIPTIONISTS

I asked some successful medical transcriptionists, "What do you have to say to someone considering a career in medical transcription?" Here's what they said:

Marcy Diehl, CMT, is probably the best known medical transcription educator in the country. She is author of the most widely used medical transcription textbook, as well as numerous other books and articles. She has a wealth of knowledge to share. Here's some of it:

> *"So! You are thinking about learning more about a medical transcription career. I am so glad that you have heard of this career and the wonderful opportunities you have available to learn more about it. To say that medical transcription is exciting and offers a life-long*

challenge to those with a keen interest in medicine, is not giving it its due. There is just so much more. But if you like a challenge, if you love words and the wonderful way they are strung together (and separated), if sitting at a computer terminal is attractive to you, then learn more! Learn more about the field; learn where you can best obtain your training; learn to know when you are ready to begin your career; and learn how to get started performing the art of medical transcription."

Gerri Dunham, CMT, is past president of the San Diego Chapter of the AAMT and supervises the medical transcription department of a local hospital. She is very encouraging to those interested in the profession, and likes to invite them to visit her department. Gerri says:

"Medical transcription is a fascinating, rewarding, as well as humbling profession. In the future, much more technology will be required, and I would suggest more in-depth knowledge of "programming," as I believe this will be beneficial. The future appears to be very good for medical transcription, even in the day of the "voice recognition systems" we hear so much about. There will always be the need for "hu-

man" input. Also, with so many people desiring to work from their home environment, the trend today is for "off-site" transcriptionists or independent medical transcriptionist contractors.

My suggestions would be to be involved in the best medical transcription courses that can be found; to follow up with as much information from AAMT and local AAMT chapters; to network with "experienced" transcriptionists now for their outlook on the future of medical transcription and gain from their past and present work situations. Develop a library of medical transcription reference materials."

Anita Hill, CMT, has run a very successful medical transcription service for a number of years. She also finds the time to be active in our professional association as past president of our local chapter and current treasurer of the state chapter. She has mentored many graduate students in their transition to becoming successful medical transcriptionists.

What would I say to someone considering a career in medical transcription? I would first advise that person to prepare a list of questions regarding what it is really like in the field and present that list to as many people in the profession as possible. Do careful research and select a reputable school that is not in it only for the money. It is not as easy to learn as some would have you believe; the road to success is long and full of hard work, but once you become proficient, it is a wonderful profession in which you never stop learning and where you will feel part of a team.

Strive to get to a level in transcription where you understand and can see the whole picture of a report. This is important in picking up mistakes the doctors often make, such as left/ right and "gender benders," as well as what medication treats what disease; some of them sound so similar but treat different illnesses. I look at this as having arrived at a certain level of expertise.

I would further advise that person to "team up" with a mentor; not to "get a job," but to have support and guidance along the way. It is, of course, also very important to belong to the professional organization(s) of medical tran-

**HARRISON COUNTY
PUBLIC LIBRARY**
105 North Capitol Ave.
Corydon, IN 47112

scription where mentors are available and
which gives one a "bay view window" and a
"finger on the pulse" of this profession, includ-
ing information on new books, job openings,
national services, new technology, where and
when important meetings are held, etc., etc.
When subsequently working, I would advise the
person to consider becoming a mentor for
someone new in the field.

Jennifer Martin somehow manages to teach, produce a
very successful newsletter, and raise a family. Yet she
remains one of the most active, cheerful, enthusiastic,
knowledgeable, and helpful people in the business. Here's
what she has to say to you:

Medical transcription is a skilled profession. It
is not a business that will make you an over-
night success. It does pay well — after you have
put some time and energy into learning it. As
your skills improve, so will your income.

Look into every available avenue as far as
education, including local college courses and
independent study programs. Talk to medical
office managers, transcription service owners

HARRISON COUNTY
PUBLIC LIBRARY

and hospital transcription supervisors. Start
networking now — that is how 90% of you will
find your first job. Good luck!

Stella Olson, CMT, is past president of AAMT, a successful business owner highly respected in the business community, a consultant, and dynamo. She has these words for you:

> *"Anyone considering to become a medical*
> *transcriptionist today should look at this on a*
> *long-range basis. It is important to know that*
> *we are a changing profession, as well as society,*
> *and technology plays a very important role in*
> *our future. To become a medical transcription-*
> *ist today means that you are the medical*
> *information specialist of tomorrow——far*
> *beyond the keyboard. Approach your new*
> *profession with the attitude of continued*
> *learning as long as you are in the field; it will*
> *take you to broader and bigger heights."*

Gayle Vindiola, CMT, was in one of my classes not so
long ago. Now she's a Certified Medical Transcriptionist and
president-elect of our local AAMT chapter. I would like to
pass her enthusiasm along to you.

> *I never would have thought that I could sit in*
> *front of a computer for eight hours or more a*

*day typing. As it turns out, I love what I do, I'm
never bored, and the time goes by very quickly.
I became a CMT after working only two and a
half years for a transcription service.*

Adrienne Yazidjian, CMT, is a another success story.
She's done everything! She is past president of AAMT. She
formed her own medical transcription service, which became
very successful and was recently bought by one of the large
national services.

*Briefly stated, if you enjoy being a word detec-
tive, can recognize, evaluate and interpret
discrepancies in the spoken word, have good
command of the English language in general,
have the ability to use reference materials, love
a challenge, and can set goals for yourself on an
hourly basis with regard to production, enjoy
seeing a perfect finished product, are detail-
oriented, can keep up with new trends and
developments in medicine, will document revised
and new terminology, styles and definitions for
reference and application, are ready for (or have
already learned about) life with new technology, meaning PC environment, then you are on
the road to an exciting professional career as a
medical transcriptionist.*

You'll hear many more words of welcome and encourage-ment as you network with the strong, supportive, and suc-cessful members of the medical transcription community.

An interview with a medical transcriptionist

It seems like only yesterday that **Lyn Gard, CMT**, was a student of mine. Now she's a certified medical transcriptionist and running a successful home business with as much work as she can handle. I'm sure you can sense her enthusiasm.

Q: Why did you choose medical transcription as a career?

Lyn: After many years in publishing, it was no longer stimu-lating. With a gift for language, and being fast on the keyboard, I thought that my skills would be well suited to a more interesting career in medical transcription.

Q: With this background, was it easy to train?

Lyn: It was NOT easy. I had to work hard and study hard. I had the time to take an intensive program, and eventu-ally got into a work experience situation offered by the college, where I went out to a work site as part of my training.

Q: Was this work experience class useful?

Lyn: Oh yes. "This is fun," I thought. "Can I do more?" Luckily, there was still a second work experience situation available, so I was working in two different medical transcription offices as part of my education. After a year of intensive school work, I was hired as a medical transcriptionist by one of those employers.

Q: Were you ready, after all that education?

Lyn: I still had a lot to learn. Even now I'm still learning. The medical transcriptionist is always learning. My first employer was an excellent mentor, taking time to proofread my work at first, until gradually I was able to work unsupervised. Now I've started my own medical transcription service, where I have my own clients, but sometimes I help her out with her overload.

Q: Describe your home office.

Lyn: It's cozy! You don't need to spend a lot of money to get started. I'm building up my equipment as I go along. I managed to get a used dictation system, which is basically a telephone answering machine where my doctors can call in and dictate their reports onto cassette tapes. I manage fine with just one incoming line for dictation. I don't have a digital recording system yet. I have four different transcribers to play back the cassettes. I have a "C-phone," which is just a little box of electronics that allows my phone to connect to an outside dictation system, so I don't have to physically collect tapes from someone else's office. And of course, a modem is essential in this business.

Q: Is it important to get some outside experience before setting up your home business?

Lyn: Absolutely. No matter how intensive your education was, you need a lot of practical experience before you can go "independent." It's not easy.

Q: Why did you go for CMT certification?

Lyn: CMT certification is a symbol of our professionalism. It's a challenge. Something to work hard for. It shows you and employers that you're good at what you do, and that you want to be better. It's something to live up to.

Q: Do you enjoy your work?

Lyn: Immensely! I'm crazy about it. It's a true career. In medical transcription, I chose the right path. It's a very flexible career. As a medical transcriptionist, I feel that eventually I will be able to "cruise" into my retirement, and work at this part-time. I'll be able to adjust my work hours to suit my lifestyle and my location. I'm very happy with it.

SAMPLE
MEDICAL REPORTS

SAMPLE MEDICAL REPORT # 1

PULMONARY CONSULTATION

Reason for Consultation: Pneumonia.

Present Illness: This 81-year-old lady has apparently
enjoyed good health most of her life. Apparently she had
been taking some "water pill" for her hypertension, but
otherwise had been on no regular medication. In fact, aside
from cataract surgery, she has not required hospitalization in
the past.

Apparently, about a week ago, she fell at home and sus-
tained an injury, presumably to her pelvis, although the
patient's son is not exactly sure of the nature of her injury.
She was evaluated by Dr. Jones and was started on Tylenol
with codeine, as well as meprobamate. For the last week, the
patient has been at home and spent much of her time in bed.
There is no apparent history of aspiration or nausea or
vomiting.

Early this morning, the patient was found by her husband
to be confused and complaining of trouble catching her

breath. The paramedics were summoned and she was brought to the Anytown Hospital emergency room. In the emergency room, she was found to be lethargic but with stable vital signs. When the history was obtained, she was given two ampules of Narcan and apparently became much more responsive.

A chest film, however, was taken which demonstrates an extensive right-sided pneumonia throughout the right lung. There is a question of an early infiltrate at the left base as well. Initial arterial blood gases done in the emergency room showed pO_2 44 and pCO_2 40, with pH 7.53 on room air. Electrocardiogram was unremarkable save for a rare PVC and occasional PAC's. Hemoglobin was 11.3 and white count 11,100 with a shift to the left, 35 polys and 54 bands.

According to the patient's son, there is no prior history of lung disease. There is no history of chronic dyspnea or cough. The patient herself is still somewhat confused and doesn't give a very coherent history. She, however, denies dyspnea, cough, or hemoptysis at this time. Apparently there has been no history of chest pain. The patient is a non-smoker.

Past Medical History: Medications as noted above. Allergies: None known. Previous hospitalizations: Only for cataract surgery.

Review of Systems: HEENT: Negative. Cardiac: No history of chest pain, heart murmur, or rheumatic fever.

History of hypertension as noted above. Pulmonary: See Present Illness. GI: No history of abdominal pain, hematemesis, melena, or jaundice. GU: No history of dysuria or hematuria. Musculoskeletal: No history of arthritis or muscle weakness. Neurologic: No history of seizures or syncope. Endocrine: No history of diabetes or goiter. No history of weight loss.

Family History: Noncontributory.

Social History: Noncontributory.

Physical Examination: General appearance: This is an elderly white female who is oriented only to person, but is otherwise in no distress. Vital signs: Temperature 100.6 degrees, respiratory rate 20, pulse 88, blood pressure 130/80. Skin: Unremarkable. Head: Atraumatic. EENT: Sclerae white, conjunctivae pink, fundi benign. Throat is negative. Ear canals are not examined. Neck is supple without jugular venous distention or thyroid enlargement. Chest: There are coarse early to mid-inspiratory crackles heard at the left base as well. No wheezes are appreciated. Heart: The PMI is within the midclavicular line. S1 and S2 are normal. An S4 gallop is heard. A II/VI systolic murmur is heard at the apex with some radiation to the axilla. Abdomen: Normal bowel sounds. No hepatosplenomegaly or other masses. There is a well-healed surgical scar apparently from the cesarean section. Extremities show trace pedal edema. There is evidence of chronic venous insufficiency but no signs of phlebitis. There is no clubbing or cyanosis. Screening neurologic examination is within normal limits except for the disorientation.

Assessment: The patient has a rather extensive pneumonia. There is nothing in her history to suggest aspiration. Presumably she was predisposed to the pneumonia secondary to her fall and lying down in bed. Her lethargy is probably a combination of hypoxemia and the use of tranquilizers and codeine.

My suggestions in the hospital would be to obtain appropriate sputum and blood cultures and then start her on a broad-spectrum antibiotic, such as Ancef. Supplemental oxygen will be administered, and she will be begun on a brief program of respiratory therapy.

Thank you very much for asking us to participate in this lady's care.

SAMPLE MEDICAL REPORT #2

ABDOMINAL ECHOGRAM

History: Abdominal pain, hematuria.

Procedure: Multiple real-time images through the liver demonstrate homogeneous transmission without bile duct dilatation or mass. The aorta is not dilated. Gallbladder is normal in position and configuration without wall thickening or stones. The common bile duct is 3 mm in diameter.

Pancreas is normal in position and configuration. Right kidney measures 12.0 x 5.5 cm, with slight calyceal dilatation. Left kidney measures 11.0 x 5.0 cm, without mass or hydronephrosis, and the spleen is 10 cm in greatest dimension.

Impression:

1. Slight infundibulocalyceal dilatation on the right, of uncertain clinical significance.

2. Otherwise echographically negative examination of the abdomen, gallbladder, and kidneys.

INTRAVENOUS PYELOGRAM

History: Hematuria. Positive family history for renal tumor.

The preliminary radiograph of the abdomen is negative.

Procedure: Following injection of 100 cc of Renografin-60, there is prompt excretion bilaterally in the nephrographic phase. The renal contours are normal, including tomographic sections. Each ureter drains readily to the urinary bladder, which is normally distensible. There is a moderately enlarged uterus indenting the dome of the bladder. For this reason, a small mucosal-based lesion cannot be excluded. Postvoid film is unremarkable.

Impression:

1. Negative upper urinary tract.

2. Prominent uterine indentation upon the dome of the bladder. Mucosal-based lesion has not been totally excluded.

SAMPLE MEDICAL REPORT #3

PSYCHIATRIC CONSULTATION

This is the first psychiatric evaluation for a 22-year-old married mother who is a drugstore clerk. She was referred by the emergency room following the smoking of one marijuana cigarette on Saturday, June 3, probably laced with a hallucinogen such as PCP. This patient immediately had a psychotic reaction with visual hallucinations, difficulty concentrating, flashing lights, anxiety, and was seen in the emergency room, where she was given an injection of droperidol. She then developed motor restlessness and was given an injection of Benadryl, and then was sent home. Subsequently, she has been on Mellaril, 25 mg b.i.d. and h.s., and has found that although the flashing lights and visual hallucinations have resolved, she continues to be profoundly anxious with fidgetiness and motor restlessness and is extremely fearful.

The patient has not had serious physical illnesses, operations, or injuries. She denies taking any prescription medications, over-the-counter medications, prior experimentation with alcohol or drugs, but does drink quite a bit of caffeine. She does not smoke cigarettes. She had a cesarean section with the birth of her only child almost two years ago.

She is in a stable marriage, and her parents and five siblings are healthy. She has had no other major life stressors, and has had no prior psychiatric contacts.

Other than this current episode, she has never had psychosis, mania, organic brain syndrome, and has not had any episodes of suicidal or homicidal ideation. She knows of no mental illness or substance abuse history in her family.

She was seen today without her medical chart. She is obviously quite akathitic, and she was advised to discontinue taking the Mellaril and to begin taking Ativan, 2 mg q.i.d., together with Benadryl, 50 mg q.i.d. She was given a handout on minor tranquilizers. She will be supervised by her husband and will return to see me in one week.

Diagnosis:

Axis I: Psychotic organic brain syndrome secondary to hallucinogens (?PCP and marijuana).

Axis II: None.

Axis III: Akathisia secondary to droperidol and/or Mellaril.

Axis IV: Level of stressors is moderate (bad drug trip).

Axis V: Level of functioning is poor. Highest level of functioning in the past year was good.

Thank you for this interesting consultation.

SAMPLE MEDICAL REPORT #4

OPERATIVE REPORT

Preoperative Diagnosis: Esotropia.

Postoperative Diagnosis: Esotropia.

Operation: 5 mm bilateral medial rectus recession.

Anesthesia: General endotracheal inhalation.

Indications for Operation: The patient is a 10 -year-old boy with a long-standing history of esotropia. He had been patched in the past until his vision was essentially equal. He had no significant refractive error. He had a deviation measuring approximately 40 diopters of esotropia. He is admitted at this time for surgical correction of the deviation.

Operative Procedure: Under adequate general endotracheal inhalation anesthesia, both eyes and periorbita were prepped in the usual fashion. Sterile Lacri-Lube ointment was placed in the left eye, and the lids of the left eye were gently closed. The patient was then draped with the right eye exposed. A wire eyelid speculum was placed in the right eye. The 6, 12, 3, and 9 o'clock positions were marked at the limbus with a marking pen. A traction suture of #5-0 Mersilene, double-armed on a spatula needle, was then passed through conjunctiva and episclerae at the limbus at the 6 and 12 o'clock position. This traction was used to rotate the globe temporally so the area over the right medial rectus muscle was exposed. An incision was made through conjunctiva and Tenon's capsule at the limbus in the horizontal meridian, corresponding to the right medial rectus insertion. This incision was carried 1½ clock hours on either side. Relaxing incisions were made in the conjunctiva, and the relaxed conjunctiva was tagged with interrupted sutures of #7-0 Vicryl. Westcott scissors were used to bluntly dissect conjunctiva and Tenon's capsule from the underlying sclera and the infranasal and supranasal quadrants. A Jameson muscle hook was then passed behind the right medial rectus muscle. Attachments of Tenon's capsule, check ligament, and intramuscular septum to the right medial rectus muscle were dissected free from the muscle using a combination of sharp and spreading dissection with Westcott scissors, as well as blunt dissection with a damp Q-tip. In this fashion, the right medial rectus muscle was isolated from its attachments. A second Jameson muscle hook was passed behind the muscle to ensure that all the fibers of the muscle were incorporated in the hook, which indeed they were. A suture of #6-0 Vicryl, double-armed on a spatula needle, was then passed through the insertion of the muscle and double-locked in place at the superior and inferior pole. The right medial rectus muscle was then disinserted from the globe. A few small bleeders in the muscle stump were cauterized using the Malis cautery unit. A point was then measured off on the sclera 5 mm posterior to the original insertion, and the muscle was reattached to the sclera at this point, thereby effecting a 5 mm recession of the right medial rectus muscle.

When the recession had been accomplished in this fashion, the muscle was irrigated with gentamicin 40 mg/cc for a total volume of 0.33. Conjunctiva was then returned to its position at the limbus, where it was sutured in place using the preplaced sutures of #7-0 Vicryl and allowing for a 1.5 mm conjunctival recession. This essentially completed surgery on the right eye. The traction suture and the #5-0 Mersilene and the eyelid speculum were removed. Maxitrol ophthalmic ointment was then placed in the right eye, and the lids of the right eye were gently closed.

Drapes were then removed from the right eye, and a new set of drapes was placed, this time exposing the left eye. At this point in time, precisely the same procedure was performed on the left eye as just described for the right, namely a 5 mm recession of the medial rectus muscle, this time of the left medial rectus muscle. Surgery in the left eye was performed in precisely the same fashion as described for the right eye, and surgery in the left eye went smoothly and uneventfully, just as it had in the right eye. At the conclusion of surgery on the left eye, that eye also was dressed with Maxitrol ophthalmic ointment.

At the conclusion of surgery, the Maxitrol ophthalmic ointment was left as the only dressing. No patches were applied to the eyes. At the conclusion of surgery, the patient was extubated uneventfully and returned to the recovery room in good condition, having tolerated the procedure well.

SAMPLE MEDICAL REPORT #5

PATHOLOGY REPORT

Clinical Diagnosis: Carcinoma, left breast.

Tissue and Location: Tissue, left breast and axillary node.

Gross Description: 630 gm left breast with axillary tail. The skin ellipse measures 15 x 6 cm, and no skin scar is recognized grossly. The nipple measures 1 cm in diameter and is free of crust. The deep margin is inked black, and serial sections show a very well-circumscribed, faintly gritty, tan tumor mass in the upper inner quadrant measuring 2.6 x 2.5 x 2.0 cm. Tumor abuts on deep fascia. 2 gm of tumor is sent for hormone receptor analysis. Other regions of breast show fibrocystic changes. Numerous lymph nodes are identified in the axillary tail. RSx12

Cassette Summary:

1.	deep margin	8.	nipple
2-4.	tumor	9.	skin
5.	upper outer quadrant	10-12.	nodes
6.	lower outer quadrant	R1.	additional deep margin
7.	lower inner quadrant		

Microscopic: Sections show a very well-circumscribed tumor comprised of cells with large hyperchromatic nuclei and abundant eosinophilic cytoplasm. Some features indicate medullary carcinoma, such as the well-circumscribed border, predominant syncytial growth pattern, and faint but present lymphoplasmacytic infiltrate. On the other hand, some features argue agaisnt the diagnosis of medullary carcinoma, including the rather uniform appearance of the neoplastic cells and the focal suggestion of tubule formation. In addition, other sections of breast from the upper outer quadrant show microscopic foci of abnormal intraductal epithelial cells, possibly representing ductal carcinoma in situ. In conclusion, the tumor is best interpreted as a high-grade infiltrating ductal carcinoma. Tumor is close to the deep margins in many areas, and in one microscopic focus tumor is touching the inked margin. The skin and nipple are free of tumor. A total of 14 axillary lymph nodes are all free of metastatic carcinoma.

TEST YOUR
MEDICAL TRANSCRIPTION
POTENTIAL

QUESTIONS

*T*his quiz is just for fun. There is no official score which signifies whether or not you'd make a good medical transcriptionist. Everything here can be learned. But of course, if you do well, then you're certainly a good candidate. (Answers are on page 139)

1. Do you have an interest in medicine?

2. Do you think that misspellings or bad grammar in a book, magazine article, business letter/memo are unprofessional?

3. As a medical transcriptionist, if you hear a word you don't understand, do you think it's more helpful to the dictating doctor if you guess at the word rather than leave a blank space?

4. As a medical transcriptionist, your employer begins to place more and more emphasis on quantity of production and less on the quality. To further boost production, she drops the quality-control person who did the proofreading, and instead has that person do simply

transcription. Do you think this is good business practice on the part of your employer?

5. You are a medical transcriptionist working overtime in Dr. Smith's office one evening. You are alone. One of her patients calls and asks for his lab test results. You happen to have just transcribed that very report, and the chart is on your desk. Would you be doing everyone a favor by just giving out that information over the phone?

6. Do you think continuing education is important for the medical transcriptionist? If so, why? If not, why not?

7. Which of the following sentences is incorrectly punctuated?

    a) The children's toys were scattered around the waiting room.

    b) The ICU was filled to its capacity.

    c) After only two hours of treatment, the blood pressure was back to normal.

    d) In one weeks time, the cast can be removed.

8. Below are some very commonly misspelled words. One of each pair is correct. Which?

accommodate	accomodate
siezure	seizure
inflamation	inflammation
inflamed	inflammed
physciatry	psychiatry
definate	definite
possession	posession
perscription	prescription

9. b.i.d., t.i.d., and q.i.d. are terms that tell how many times in a day a medication should be taken. How many times a day does each term mean? (Clue: You already know some common words with similar prefixes: e.g., bilateral, tripod, quartet, etc.)

10. Would you like to start a home-based medical transcription service within the next year?

11. What skills and characteristics do you think would make a good medical transcriptionist?

SOME MEDICAL TRANSCRIPTION RESOURCES

The American Association for Medical Transcription (AAMT), P.O. Box 576187, Modesto, CA 95357-6187. Tel. (800) 982-2182. This is a nonprofit professional association (see Chapter 9 for more information). They won't try to sell you anything. They'll be happy to answer any questions you have about medical transcription, and will send you a packet of information just for the asking. They'll give you the name of someone to contact at your local chapter. You'll be a welcome guest at local chapter meetings. There's a student rate if you decide to become a member.

MT Monthly, 1633 N.E. Rosewood Drive, Gladstone, MO 64118. Tel. (800) 951-5559. This monthly newsletter costs $48 per year. Aside from the Journal of AAMT, it is probably the most widely read (and respected) medical transcription publication, where medical transcriptionists share practical information, useful advice, and a broad range of opinions.

Advance for Health Information Professionals. Tel. (800) 355-5627. This is a biweekly publication that usually contains an interesting article or two on medical transcription. There's a good classified ads section with jobs available around the country. This publication is free.

The Independent Medical Transcriptionist, by Donna Avila-Weil and Mary Glaccum, published by Rayve Publications. When you're ready to start your own home medical transcription business, this book will be a valuable asset. Wait until then before you buy it, because technology and the medical transcription work environment are changing so fast. You'll want the most up-to-date version of this comprehensive, fact-filled, no-nonsense, hard-reality book.

http://www.mtdaily.com

If that looks like an Internet address, you're right. This is the web page for medical transcriptionists, crammed full of facts and information. No sales stuff here, although there are links to commercial sites. Don't miss it.

Home-Office Computing is an excellent monthly magazine. It's not for computer nerds but for creative and independent people in all walks of life who need to use computers. Highly recommended. It's at your local magazine stand. Subscription information at 1-800-288-7812. Their web page is at http://www.smalloffice.com

Guerrilla Marketing for Home Businesses and **Guerrilla Marketing Attack** are two of an excellent series of books by Jay Conrad Levinson. They're best-sellers and in any bookstore or library. Very well written and very inspiring. Have one of them by your side as you start your home business.

Prodigy, **Compuserve**, and **America On-Line** have forums where medical transcriptionists share advice and opinions.

The Small Business Administration has a local office listed in your phone book (U.S. Government listings), and they're on the Internet at http://sba.com

gmorton@mail.gcccd.cc.ca.us

That's my e-mail address. All questions, comments, and feedback are welcome. Please tell me what you think of this book.

TEST YOUR MEDICAL TRANSCRIPTION POTENTIAL

ANSWERS

1. If you're interested in medicine, you'll probably do a lot better as a medical transcriptionist than someone who isn't. You'll certainly enjoy it a lot more. And if you're FASCINATED by medicine, better still!

2. Misspellings and bad grammar don't always matter in casual communication. But in many business and professional situations, they're vitally important. Misspellings and bad grammar can make serious (even fatal) differences in medical reports. (See Chapter 2, Accuracy)

3. The documents produced by the medical transcriptionist are medically and legally worthless if they contain guesswords. What credence could a court of law give to such a document? No one could tell what is accurate and what is not. On the other hand, a document that contains blank spaces where words or phrases were in doubt, is still medically and legally acceptable when there is reasonable assurance that the remaining text is accurate.

4. If the quantity of your work as a medical transcriptionist is more important to your employer than its quality, then you're working for the wrong person. Substandard medical transcription is medically and legally dangerous.

5. You are wrong to divulge this information over the phone. There are a number of reasons. First, you don't even know if this is actually the patient at the other end of the line. All kinds of snoopers use this trick. Don't fall for it. Second, the medical report and the information therein belong not to the patient but to the doctor or the doctor's employer. Only the doctor has the right to divulge this information. Third, the information belongs in the context of the complete medical picture. One test result may be more or less serious according to many other factors. It is the doctor's responsibility to present this medical information to the patient in context.

6. A medical transcriptionist cannot survive without continuing education. There are new terms, new procedures, and new medications every week. You can't do this work if you don't know what the doctors are talking about! (See Chapter 2, Continuing Education)

7. (d) There is no such thing as "one weeks." This is a possessive (in the time of one week) not a plural. It should be written "one week's."

8.

accommodate	seizure
inflammation	inflamed
psychiatry	definite
possession	prescription

9. Twice a day, three times a day, and four times a day respectively.

10. There are certainly great opportunities for starting a home-based medical transcription service. But you must be realistic. It will likely take you far more than a year to reach a level of proficiency that will enable you to succeed in a competitive business. There's a lot to learn! (See Chapters 7 and 8).

11. See Chapter 3.

MEDICAL
LANGUAGE DEVELOPMENT

- Medical language education for attorneys, paralegals, insurance professionals, psychologists, and everyone involved in health care.

- Medical transcription career-information seminars

- Medical transcription education and recruitment

- Publishing

For information on any of these services, please contact

Medical Language Development
4122 Cortez Way
Spring Valley, CA 91977-1319
tel: (619) 660-9845
e-mail: gmorton@mail.gcccd.cc.ca.us

How to become a medical transcriptionist
A 653. 18 MOR   2209

Morton, George.
HARRISON COUNTY PUBLIC LIBRARY

ADDITIONAL COPIES

of

How To Become
A Medical Transcriptionist:
A Career for the 21st Century

can be ordered from

Medical Language Development

4122 Cortez Way

Spring Valley, CA 91977

tel: (619) 660-9845

e-mail: gmorton @mail.gcccd.cc.ca.us

Cost is $12.95 per book, plus $1.50 shipping.

California residents must add the appropriate sales tax

Discounts are available for larger orders.

Please inquire for details.